Stretching Exercises

Encyclopedia

Óscar Morán (author)
Isabel Arechabala (illustrations)

Stretching Exercises

Encyclopedia

Original Version by Pila Teleña; © 2009
C/ Pozo Nuevo, 12
28430 Alpedrete (Madrid)
e-mail: pilatelena@pilatelena.com

Coverdesign: Sabine Groten

British Library Cataloguing in Publication Data
A catalogue record for this book is available from the British Library

Stretching Exercises Encyclopedia
Maidenhead: Meyer & Meyer Sport (UK) Ltd., 2012
ISBN 978-1-84126-351-9

© 2012 by Meyer & Meyer Sport (UK) Ltd.
Auckland, Beirut, Budapest, Cairo, Cape Town, Dubai, Indianapolis,
Kindberg, Maidenhead, Sydney, Olten, Singapore, Tehran, Toronto
Member of the World
Sport Publishers' Association (WSPA)
www.w-s-p-a.org
Printed by: B.O.S.S Druck und Medien GmbH
ISBN 978-1-84126-351-9
E-Mail: info@m-m-sports.com
www.m-m-sports.com

Contents

Acknowledgements

Isabel Arechabala
Fernando Barral
Felipe Casanueva
Marta Gil
Carmen López
Javier Morán
Marco Pila
Ewa Szczerba

My appreciation and gratitude to all of them, who have demonstrated great professionalism in the poses for this book.

Introduction

The human body is, if one can forgive the expression, tremendously conservative. People, like most living creatures, are designed to feed, reproduce and avoid danger. All energy expenditures beyond these basic abilities are unusual among those beings who are less developed than us, from an intelligence point of view. However, as we move up in the evolutionary chain, we find movements designed for socializing, enjoyment, etc. If human beings do not need to stretch in order to carry out their daily lives, they may possibly not find the need to do so. But, if they do not stretch, with the passing of time, their bodies will become clumsier, more painful, incapable, etc. It is of no use to look at oneself in the mirror and not stop asking the reasons why, one needs to exercise or stretch, until one feels "in shape" again. This feeling of being in good shape is so imperceptible that one only becomes aware of it once it has been lost. Therefore, the smart thing to do is to not abandon it.

Turning to nature once again, if we look at the animals, we find that they perform stretches routinely. Some of the better "athletes" in the animal world — like cats — do so very frequently, and they maintain their bodies ready for hunting and to avoid becoming prey to others.

In most of today's societies, human beings do not need to be in such good shape to survive, and the abilities of mobility are the first to be detrimentally affected by the sedentary lifestyle. However, in addition to making people more efficient at the physical level, which implies better athletic performance in some cases and a greater capacity to perform the activities of daily living in others, this book will show how regular stretching also has an effect upon the health and well-being of the individual.

Unfortunately, stretching has been largely forgotten by the people who exercise, whether regularly or sporadically. The reason could be the few aesthetic effects that are derived from its practice, at least compared to strength and resistance training, which mold the body's figure in a much more dramatic way. In modalities such as yoga, the stretches are the base and philosophy of its very essence; in dance, they are an essential complement; but in the practice of sports, they are usually reduced to a few seconds before and after the performance of the sport in question, and sometimes not even that. However, what many people don't realize is that a more agile and "flexible" body is also more proportioned from an aesthetic point of view and, as we have pointed out before, it is also more healthy.

In the book *Muscle Exercises Encyclopedia* (Morán, 2012) from the same publishing company, it is pointed out that a kyphotic posture (commonly called "hunchback"), in many cases, is caused by a lack of tone in the muscles of the back (dorsal, lumbar, etc.) combined with a hypertonicity and lack of flexibility of the anterior muscle (abdominal, pectoral, etc.). This is just an example of how a well-balanced body also needs to be flexible.

After reading this book, any athlete, and even those who are not athletes, will realize how regular stretching can improve their physical body shape and their quality of life.

How to use this book

All readers, regardless of their degree of mobility or their knowledge of the subject, will find an interest in this book. This is a reference manual where, with the help of the index, the reader can turn to any page in order to learn how to perform an exercise.

The pictures that accompany the text are of real professional models who were trained to perform the exercises and supervised by the author of this book.

Each exercise includes information about the movement one needs to perform, the posture that one must adopt, common mistakes that should be avoided, the principal and secondary muscles worked with this exercise, as well as a series of very useful tips and advice.

How to interpret the exercise cards

- **Name**. Most of the stretching exercises lack a common name, and so in this text they are named according to the purpose of the movement or the posture.

- **Ilustration**. The position, correct movement of the basic exercise, and the muscles involved will be shown in a drawing in "anatomical position" (only the principal and the superficial muscles involved).

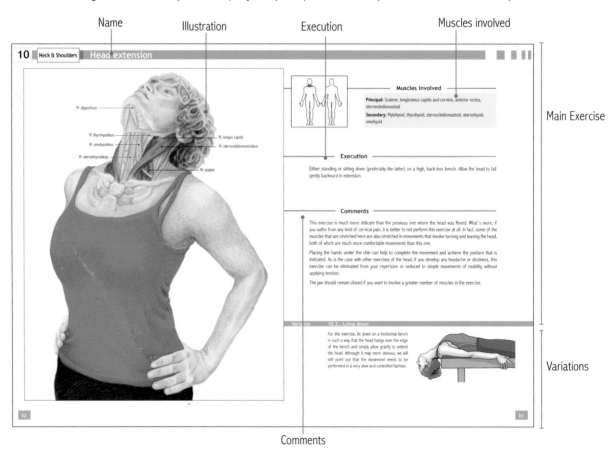

- **Muscles involved**. Named according to their order of importance in the exercise, although this order may vary depending on slight adjustments in posture or the specific characteristics of the individual person. Some muscles that are exercised only slightly have been omitted.

- **Execution**. The manner in which the exercise is to be performed and the final posture that must be adopted.

- **Comments**. Explanations, tips and common mistakes to avoid.

- **Variations**. Some exercises are complemented with certain variations. In other cases additional explanations and tips are given to the interested reader.

- **Biomechanical introduction to the principal muscles**. Given the practical nature of this book, this section, which precedes every chapter, includes a brief anatomical review of the points of origin and insertion, as well as the function of the principal muscles (whether because of their size or the role they play). This section refers to general human characteristics, which may vary in some cases depending on the individual.

Theory of Muscle Stretching

It is a good idea to begin the study of stretches by clearing up several different concepts that are related but not equivalent. *Stretching* refers to the action and effect of stretching, and we can define stretch as elongating or dilating something, pulling it apart by force so that it gives of itself; it is just like spreading or moving our arms or legs to warm them up and get the stiffness out. *Flexibility* is, on the other hand, the ability to bend easily.

Of the four basic physical qualities (also called abilities, although the author prefers the traditional term) in humans: flexibility, strength, resistance and speed; stretches are included in the first of them.

Stretches have been studied and taught by some of the most important authors in history, such as Ling, Buck, Medau, etc. Around the middle of the 20th century, some authors in the field of neurophysiology spread the technique of contraction-relaxation in the stretching exercises. This marked the beginning of Proprioceptive Neuromuscular Facilitation (P.N.F.) and the modern *stretching* that was popularized by Bob Anderson and others of the time.

This book is a compendium of exercises based on the various theories of physical training in general, and flexibility in particular.

How to stretch

There is a belief concerning stretching exercises that, if there is no pain, there is no gain. What´s more, some advocate movements that cause pain in and of themselves, very close to the limits of the joints and ligaments. Other theories recommend bouncing to achieve more and more lengthening.

This author belongs to a different school of thought, the one that promotes a rational, scientifically proven and effective stretching. It is called *stretching* in many languages, an anglicized term that comprises a global concept of stretches. The theory of the stimulus thresholds in physical exercise is also valid in stretching. This can be easily understood with the following examples:

- A stretch that is too light will produce almost no effect upon the organism, nor any improvement in joint mobility.

- A stretch that is too violent or too extreme could cause an injury, or in the best of cases, a protective muscular contracture that could prevent you from improving your flexibility.

- A stretch that is just right, forcing mobility but without reaching pain or the limits of danger, will not only be more bearable, but it also produces better results. A stretch that is just right means more than the muscle is subjected to in everyday life, demanding, but not injurious.

With most physical activity, at least in those of certain intensity, the warm-up is imperative. Stretching is no exception. Some people mistake stretching with warming up, and it is not infrequent to hear some occasional athlete, or even sports journalists, comment that someone is "warming up" when what that person is actually doing is stretching. In fact, the correct thing to do is to first warm up and then stretch. The general warm-up increases blood flow and elevates the body temperature, two beneficial effects when it comes to performing physical exercise; furthermore, the specific warm-up increases the amount of blood that reaches the tissues we are about to stretch, thereby nourishing and oxygenating them.

We could review all the different stretching techniques and point out the strengths and weaknesses of each, but the reader will appreciate that we focus on those which have been proven effective, and here´s how to perform them:

1. Begin with a light aerobic activity that gets the blood flowing. You can choose to jog, ride a stationary bike, etc., for 5 to 10 minutes.

2. Perform joint movements for the area that we are going to work, as well as for adjacent areas, for 2 to 3 minutes.

3. Occasionally, perform some resistance movements of the target muscles. For example, flexing movements for the pectoral muscles on the floor or against a wall if you will be stretching this muscle afterward.

The passive warm-up, such as sitting in a sauna before exercising, does not appear to be the best or the most effective way to warm up. It is true that the outside temperature has an influence in the optimization of the stretching sessions, but the real warm-up must come from the body´s internal structures. The simple repeated flexion and extension of a joint improves the quality and degree of a subsequent flexibility exercise.

This is the moment to begin stretching, and here comes one of the most important pieces of advice from this book: the stretch should be gentle and controlled, taking it to the point of desired resistance and holding it there for a few seconds. One must avoid bouncing, ballistic movements ("throwing" the body part in question, which could result in an injury), and harmful over-exertions. The help of a partner can be very useful, but he must be knowledgeable enough and never force beyond the threshold of normal movement.

The respiration should be slow and rhythmic, generally breathing out at the same time one stretches in order to disarm the column formed by the intrathoracic-abdominal pressure. The body, and in particular the body part being stretched, must not be under excessive tension, which explains why some athletes injure themselves after practicing their sport when they conclude their training with rough stretches. And they do not understand how it is they got injured "if they were warmed up."

And what about the sedentary people who have decided to begin stretching as part of their overall plan to improve their physical health? Some sound advice is to first strengthen the body, that is, first develop a certain degree of strength, and then begin to stretch without abandoning the strength training.

And what about those periods of inactivity when you have already performed some physical exercise for a while? This is a somewhat delicate topic and one that does not present itself in all the specialties in the same way. A resistance athlete who is subjected to a period of inactivity, and then intends to take it up again, will note how his personal benchmarks are worse, both in terms of the speed sustained as well as in the total time supported. But there is no major problem; the body and its aerobic resistance will know how to dose it. In the case of stretching, as is the case with the strength training, there is a risk in wanting to recover too quickly and get back to the lifts that we were able to do before the layoff, and the uneasiness of the time away could expose one to injury. One must not fall prey to feelings of regret and frustration, but instead, one must plan intelligently, setting multiple small goals that will soon give us back the level of performance that we desire. If the inactivity has lasted too long, it is easier to recover than to start from the beginning since, although for us it may feel like a very long time, in reality it does not take that long.

There is however, one great difficulty, especially among beginners: knowing the difference between pain and discomfort. The first tends to involve a sharp and unbearable sensation, while the latter tends to be a pulling sensation resulting from the stretching. The pain does not go away even when we relax the posture, but the discomfort usually gets better when we manage to concentrate enough to overcome it.

Types of stretches

In order to stretch properly, it is necessary to know several different types of stretches, and in this way, one would be able to exercise based on his needs and objectives. We will talk about static, dynamic and PNF, but we will only detail the steps of the two methods that have been selected for their efficacy and simplicity will be discussed in detail.

—**Static stretching:** It is also referred to as passive stretching, although the two are not exactly equal. The static stretch consists of taking a joint close to the limit of its mobility and maintaining that posture for a few seconds. It is one of the simplest and most effective stretches, and we can subdivide it in two:

(i) **Active Static:** when the person stretching is the one who exerts, through the help of the other muscle groups, the force required to maintain the posture. It is not the most effective because it is not easy to maintain the proper tension for some of the body parts, and thus it is often preferable to perform passive static stretches, as explained below.

(ii) **Passive Static:** when a machine or another person helps to maintain the stretching posture. It consists of the following:

1. Stretch slowly until the limit prior to the pain.

2. Hold that position for approximately 20 seconds.

3. Pause for around 20 or 30 seconds (during which time you may stretch a different muscle group, preferably the antagonist).

4. Repeat the process 3 or 4 times.

—Dynamic Stretching: As the name implies, one takes a body part in controlled movement until reaching its maximum point. This is a type of stretching that is reserved, almost always, to certain sports modalities in which an excellent control of mobility, in all its amplitude, is necessary (the most common examples are the martial arts and dance). In any case, this type of stretching should only be practiced by people with a certain level of training and control in their movements, not beginners. This type of stretching can be subdivided into two categories:

—Explosive or ballistic stretching: This is a dynamic stretch that uses the inertia of the movement to take the joint farther than the normal range of motion. It is potentially injurious, which is why it generally should be avoided.

—Guided stretching: This involves performing the movement in a controlled fashion at all times but over a large degree of amplitude.

—Propioceptive Neuromuscular Facilitation (P. N. F.)

The PNF concept — some authors refer to it as isometrics — quite possibly derives from the North American authors Kabat, Levine and Bobath (in fact, it is also referred to as the "Kabat Method"), who made significant progress with this technique. Given that this method is a little more involved, it is meant for experienced individuals, not beginners. It consists of the following:

1. Begin with a light stretch until the point of discomfort.

2. Isometrically contract the stretched muscle for 6 to 8 seconds.

3. Relax the contraction for 2 or 3 seconds but without changing the posture.

4. Stretch a few more degrees of motion and hold the new position for 10 seconds.

5. Contract the muscle and repeat the process once or twice more.

This is a good stretching method provided that it is performed correctly. This technique is very similar to the Michell technique, in which, from the position of a stretched muscle, isometric contractions are performed, followed by a period of relaxation. At the end of each contraction, the stretch is increased a little more in search of a new motion barrier.

Smart stretching

In the stretching exercises, although it may not seem obvious to a beginner, the muscle is far from remaining passive. When we stretch a muscle, it reacts in an opposing manner to hold on to the joint and, in and of itself, this is a very important, natural and necessary mechanism to avoid sustaining injuries in our daily lives. When we add bouncing, balancing or pulling, this reflex is accentuated, making the exercise more difficult. It is called the "myotic reflex." This reflex is incredibly useful, and it prevents a joint from being stretched to its limit and thus breaking unconsciously. It is so powerful that in some cases it can manage to dislocate the joint. A clear example is what occurs during traffic accidents, particularly in sudden, unexpected accidents. When the occupant in a vehicle receives an impact upon the vehicle, the body tenses up as a protective mechanism. The majority of the joints return to their normal state in just a few seconds, but some of them, such as the neck, can suffer such a strong muscle pull that it may produce a cervical sprain, caused by the reflexive pull instead. This enormous tension is understandable if we think about the importance of the structures that they are protecting: the neck and the head.

A smart stretch must be controlled, gentle and continuous.

But it is not only the muscles that are stretched, although they are in fact the biggest protagonists. The entire joint structure is stretched. In fact, some studies confirm that certain muscles may be stretched to almost twice their normal length without injury, but other structures cannot be so easily moved. In this way, the amplitude of the movement of the joints depends on an equilibrium complex between stability and mobility. The ligaments, muscle fascias, joint capsules and especially the tendons, are compromised during the stretching exercises. When one of these structures is stretched beyond its threshold of resistance, it suffers damage, as is the case with sprains.

Smart stretching takes the joint to a point close to its limits, and so a certain amount of discomfort is normal while performing them. When this discomfort becomes pain, then we may have exceeded said limit, and we may be getting dangerously close to an injury. At the opposite extreme is the excessively lax joint, where movements are easily taken beyond the normal limits. It is at the halfway point that one finds virtue and balance. Following the stretching movement, the tension partially gives way after 3 or 4 seconds (without moving, the posture has become more pleasant), and that is a good indication that you are doing things right.

One not-so-smart stretch is that which forces a joint beyond its capabilities, which produces bouncing, or forces a muscle to hold a specific posture at the same time it pretends to stretch it (such as "standing up straight, flexing the torso with knees straight, trying to touch the ground").

Finally, it is necessary to point out a dominant factor in obtaining a good stretch: concentration. While this factor is necessary in the performance of many different sports, in stretching it is absolutely necessary. The person who stretches must concentrate on the area being stretched, and he cannot be distracted in conversations with his stretching partner, television or other things. A person who is distracted will have great difficulty in reaching the optimum stretching point, and if he falls short then the session will not have been very productive, and if he overdoes it, he may injure himself. Furthermore, in order to be able to concentrate and feel the muscles being stretched, it is necessary to have a certain knowledge of anatomy.

The moments and times for stretching

Regular athletes are not all the same when it comes to planning their stretching exercises. Some do it as part of their warm-up, others do it in the rest periods between their sets, after their training or competition is over, or even during times that are totally isolated from their regular athletic activities. What is the correct way to plan stretching? It appears that there is no single correct answer.

From all the different options presented, we could plan two basic models of stretching:

Warm-up – Stretch – Athletic activity – Stretch

Warm-up – Stretch

In the first option, stretching is presented as both a preparation for and a recuperation from the practice of physical exercise itself. In the second option, the stretching "is the physical exercise," meaning this is a session focused on stretching. There is only one exception to stretching without warming up, and that is the stretching done to get the stiffness out of the body resulting from prolonged postures at work or during the course of daily living, although that is more the case of exercises of joint mobility that are not performed for the purpose of improving the degree of flexibility.

Anyone who wishes to maintain an acceptable degree of joint mobility should stretch at least 3 to 7 times a week in sessions lasting approximately 15 minutes. Yet if the goal is to actually improve – not just maintain – flexibility, then these stretching sessions should be increased to 5 or 6 times a week and last from 15 to 30 minutes each. Among the elite athletes, whose sport practices demand tremendous joint mobility from them (for example, some types of gymnastics), the time dedicated specifically to stretching is generally more than one hour per day and it is done every day of the week.

Each exercise described in this book should be repeated between 3 and 6 times, holding each of them for approximately 10 to 20 seconds. It is better to stretch almost all of the muscles during each stretching session rather than divide them into separate muscle groups on different days (as is the case with strength training). To avoid getting tired of the routine and to not leave body parts un-stretched, it is a good idea to change the exercises chosen each week. If pressed for time, you may divide the body in two and do the exercises corresponding to each of the 2 areas of the body on alternate days.

During the short rest periods in the stretching sessions, we can stretch the antagonistic muscle group. For example, if you are stretching the quadriceps, in the rest periods between consecutive sets you could stretch the hamstrings. This is useful for making up time and for not leaving any areas of the body un-stretched.

Even though this book praises the stretching exercises performed to improve flexibility, the author would like to put in its proper place the importance of this quality. It is not true that it is equally beneficial to all sports; it's logical to think that a gymnast or a martial artist will need more flexibility than a sprinter. The first two will dedicate a great part of their training to improving their joint mobility, whereas the latter will spend much more time improving his aerobic resistance. To do otherwise would be counterproductive to their sports performance. What´s more, excessive flexibility training can reduce the efficiency of other physical qualities, such as strength. Lastly, while it is true that flexibility training prevents some types of injuries, the majority of these may be suffered whether one has good flexibility or not. So it cannot be said that a flexible person has a "much lower risk" of injury than someone who is not as flexible, especially if his chosen athletic activities do not challenge the limits of joint mobility. Flexibility training is necessary, but the most important thing is to do it in the proper amount.

Place and conditions for stretching

Unlike other physical exercises, stretching does not require any machines, special attire or special equipment. It is enough to simply wear conventional athletic clothing and a mat in case the floor is too hard. However, group stretching and some of the equipment that is found in the gym may favor or improve your stretching, whether it is by improving motivation or by other means.

The environment should be warm, not just in terms of temperature, but also from an emotional or psychological perspective. If there is music, it is preferable that it be slow and relaxing.

The practice of stretching exercises in nature is particularly gratifying. The woods, the beach, the grass in a city park... are all ideal places for stretching. Unlike other sporting activities, stretching requires a high degree of internalizing, and if the environment matches, the results are better.

But these practices are not limited to just scheduled times, whether in a gym or somewhere else. Any daily activity, whether it is during work, study, etc., can be interrupted for a few minutes to practice some stretches. Those who do, so attest that their "batteries are recharged" after they stretch, they feel better physically, and they are ready to perform better when they return to their activities.

Regarding clothing, the recommendations are similar to those for other physical activities; that is, you should wear athletic clothing that is light, breathable, and does not constrain the body. It should not have any bothersome seams, rivets or metal pieces. The footwear is not as important as it is with other athletic activities, and in fact, the majority of the stretching exercises may be performed barefoot or wearing socks. The only difference that should be noted is that, for stretching, it is preferable that the clothing covers most of the body and provides some warmth; that is, it is better to feel a little hot than to perform the exercises wearing a pair of shorts. The temperature is an ally of stretching exercises, both for improving performance and for reducing the risk of injury. But at no point should you wear those plastic outfits (or the like) that increase sweating but hinder natural temperature regulation.

Stretching in pairs

In most athletic activities, when one is not knowledgeable enough about what one is doing, there is a risk of having an accident or suffering an injury. This is just the same when it comes to stretching exercises, but when we stretch in pairs, there is a portion of the activity we do not control and which relies on the knowledge and experience of our stretching partner. Therefore, there are certain guidelines that should be followed which, in addition to preventing injuries, optimize the work and the results. Here are a few of them:

- It is necessary for both partners to know each other and exchange impressions, they should communicate adequately and know the physical shape and the limits of each other.

- The best results are obtained with pairs who are of similar height, weight and physical shape, and who share similar goals.

- Since it is difficult to know the precise moment to stop when one is stretching another person, it is imperative to establish a gesture between the two that tells the person doing the stretching not to take the movement any further. It can be a slap on the ground or something similar.

- Before beginning a stretch, both partners must know and agree between themselves as to what exercise is to be performed and up to what point it will be performed.

- If the general rule in individual stretches is the slowness of movement, this is even more so when it comes to stretching in pairs. Any movement that is "not slow" will trigger a defensive contraction reflex in the other person and prevent any proper stretching.

- When stretching in pairs, it is imperative that the holds and manipulations by the other person be performed with respect, both physical and moral.

- One must try to make the partner´s respiration natural and comfortable.

- Given that concentration is important, outside noises and conversation should be limited to the bare minimum.

- The person who is receiving the stretch should trust his partner, otherwise the individual will remain tense and this will prevent any progress.

Practically all the areas of the body may be stretched individually, but working in pairs always provides a little extra motivation, which undoubtedly will lead to improvement and continuing with the training.

Stretching and pregnancy

Some women who practice sports regularly immediately abandon all exercise as soon as they find out they are pregnant. This is not entirely appropriate. However, as with strength training, if the doctor gives the green light then the majority of women are able to perform stretching exercises during a great part of their pregnancy. What is true is that you cannot stretch in the same way when you are pregnant as when you are not; there are some basic rules to follow, some of which are common to other athletic endeavors:

1. Reduce the intensity (reduce the range of motion, less sets, increase rest time, etc.).

2. Reduce the total daily training time.

3. Avoid holding your breath.

4. Do not perform exercises that put pressure on the uterus.

5. Do not perform exercises in a decubitus prone position after the first trimester.

6. Do not perform the movements right up to the limits of mobility because the hormonal changes may provoke joint instability.

7. Fluid intake and diet must be strictly controlled.

8. The last months are the most delicate during the pregnancy, and the doctor may recommend reducing or suspending all physical exercise.

9. Avoid exercises that involve a difficult technique or are dangerous.

10. Eliminate competitive sporting activities.

11. Pay special attention to the body temperature and the temperature in the room.

12. Be careful with hygiene, and your physical and mental health.

13. You should get up slowly after the floor exercises to avoid any problems with hypotension, which could even ead to fainting.

14. The post-partum recovery should be controlled by the doctor. Most women resume their normal exercise routine again a few weeks after the delivery, particularly if there were no complications during the pregnancy and they were in good physical shape before the pregnancy.

Some of the most stressed muscle groups during pregnancy are those in the abdominal/lumbar region. The first because of the extension it undergoes as a result of the increase in the internal diameter, and the latter to support the extra weight placed on the spine. If a woman is planning to get pregnant, these are the muscle groups that she should prioritize during her training. Likewise, they are key areas after she has given birth.

People with a disability or some limitation

One must be able to differentiate whether the factors that are limiting our movement are natural or pathological, with muscles, tendons, bones, fat, internal organs and skin included in the first.

The dictionary defines disability as the impediment or difficulty of performing the tasks that are considered routine due to an alteration of certain physical or intellectual functions. The doctor and the interested person are the ones capable of deciding whether to stretch or not, or the degree to which it should be done. There are very few injuries and disabilities that prevent the performance of stretching exercises, but most of them do require certain adaptations. Let's review some of them:

- Psychological origin. Although it depends on the type and degree, in most cases it is usually enough to have a family member or another responsible individual who is knowledgeable of the situation, watch over the person´s physical and mental health. Other than that, the stretches are usually no different than in a normal training routine.

- Sensory difficulties. The blind or visually impaired, the hearing impaired and the mute can perform the same stretches as everyone else. Just in the case of training in pairs, the signals and communication must be adapted and agreed upon ahead of time between the partners. A couple of taps can be used to signal the limit of mobility and to stop applying pressure.

- Illnesses. Only the specialist physician can determine if the patient is able to do the physical training in case of illness. If the answer is yes and the patient is on medication, it is important that the doctor know the nature of the physical exercises, and that the trainer knows about the medication being taken. With stretching it is not usually that important – in the case of many illnesses – unlike with many other types of physical exercise. One of the main reasons is its lesser cardiovascular and respiratory demand and the ability to adapt the stretches to almost any physical condition.

- Difficulty in or the absence of movement in some areas of the body. There are almost always modifications available, indicated by the trainer to adapt the training to the person. One of the main advantages of this book is the enormous variety of stretching exercises that are shown, which makes it easier if one is unable to perform a particular exercise, the person can find a variant that is suitable for his / her condition.

The benefits are also in the psychological and social realms; the person feels more self-sufficient and is able to establish interpersonal relationships with his peers and training buddies: A good gym should adapt to people with disabilities, not the other way around.

With respect to injuries, generally speaking, an injury to one part of the body does not prevent stretching other parts. Furthermore, certain minor injuries, such as muscle contractures, either heal or improve tremendously with stretching exercises. Stretching, together with strength building, are indispensible in post-op recovery or after prolonged immobilization; your medical specialist will prescribe the exercises required.

Conclusion

With my students, I try to teach them that "stretching" is easy. "Stretching well" requires a certain degree of knowledge, and "stretching to improve" requires knowledge, planning and perseverance.

Throughout the previous pages, different techniques for stretching have been mentioned. Each person must choose the method and intensity, but most people will obtain results with techniques such as "static stretching" and P.N.F. after just a couple of weeks if they are consistent. Although each case is unique, stretching 3 or 4 times a week in sessions of 20 minutes may be enough. Unlike resistance strength training, where there are training routines that train a particular muscle group maybe once every 8 to 10 days, with stretching, nearly all muscle groups should be trained in every session. The order of the routine is not that important, but those parts that are lagging should be trained first, and leave the more advanced (i.e., flexible) body parts for the end of the session.

Although it is normal that all people choose their favorite stretches, it should be kept in mind that two similar stretches are not identical, and thus applying variety to your program is a way of ensuring that no body parts are left un-stretched.

The stretching exercises have a couple of drawbacks as many consider them boring, and they do not have such an effect upon the physical appearance as strength training exercises and aerobic exercises do. However, in addition to being indispensible for the optimal health of the musculoskeletal system, they do help to mold the figure and they are also prophylactic.

The first conclusion that we should draw from all of this is that stretching exercises are beneficial and necessary for all people. Furthermore, as in many other cases, it is a physical activity that must be performed with caution and the knowledge about what one is doing. The advice from the author for everyone who practices stretches is, as in other aspects of life, that they set realistic goals to keep themselves motivated. This book will help them.

Pectoral Group

Descriptive anatomy of the pectoral muscles: a biomechanical introduction to the principal muscles involved

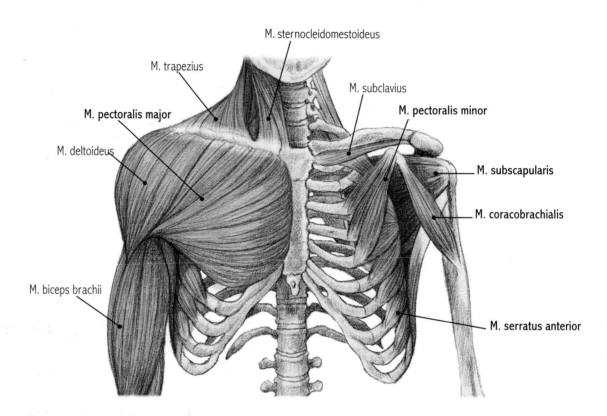

M. sternocleidomestoideus

M. trapezius

M. pectoralis major

M. deltoideus

M. biceps brachii

M. subclavius

M. pectoralis minor

M. subscapularis

M. coracobrachialis

M. serratus anterior

Muscles that insert into the humerus

Pectoral mayor (anterior, superficial)

Origin: Clavicle (clavicular portion, from the internal half of the anterior face); ribs and sternal membrane (sternocostal portion, from the cartilage); rectus abdominus (abdominal portion, from the anterior rectus sheath)

Insertion: Humerus (greater tubercular crest)

Principal functions: Anteversion of the arm if it is abducted; adduction and medial rotation; the sternocostal and abdominal portions can lower the shoulder and bring it forward; accessory muscle during inspiration (with the arm fixed)

Coracobraquial (anterior, deep)

Origin: Scapula (coracoid process)

Insertion: Humerus (medial surface, on the prolongation of the cre of the lesser tubercle)

Principal functions: Anteversion of the arm and keeping the hum ral head in the joint; assists in the adduction of the arm, dependi on the starting position

ubscapular (anterior, deep)

igin: Scapula (subscapular fossa)

sertion: Humerus (lesser tubercle and the proximal portion of its est)

incipal functions: Internal rotation of the arm

Biceps braquial (anterior, superficial)

See "BICEPS"

Brief comments: With just some basic knowledge, it is easy to stretch the pectoral muscles and the adjacent muscles, but a more careful study will make us realize that taking the proper precautions is vital in this area, as well as in others where the joint´s range of motion is significant (as is the case with the scapulo-humeral joint). Injuries involving the pectoral muscles are not uncommon, and even in the biceps, when body movements are performed right up to their limits. The pectoralis major is a strong muscle, but that does not mean that its fibers and tendon insertions can be treated with a total lack of consideration.

Muscles that do not insert into the humerus

ectoral minor (anterior, deep)

igin: Ribs (3 to 5th)

sertion. Scapula (Coracoid process)

incipal functions: Rotation and lowering of the scapula

Serratus anterior (anterior, deep)

Origin: Ribs (generally the first 9)

Insertion: Scapula (the medial border, from the superior to the inferior angle)

Principal functions: Anteversion of the arm, adhesion of the scapula to the thorax, depression and lateral rotation (lower portion), elevation (upper portion); Secondarily, elevation of the ribs (secondary muscle in respiration)

Brief comments: As in other cases, the "secondary" muscles adjacent to the pectorals are very difficult to isolate and work independently. But they receive part of the stress in the stretching exercises for the other muscles.

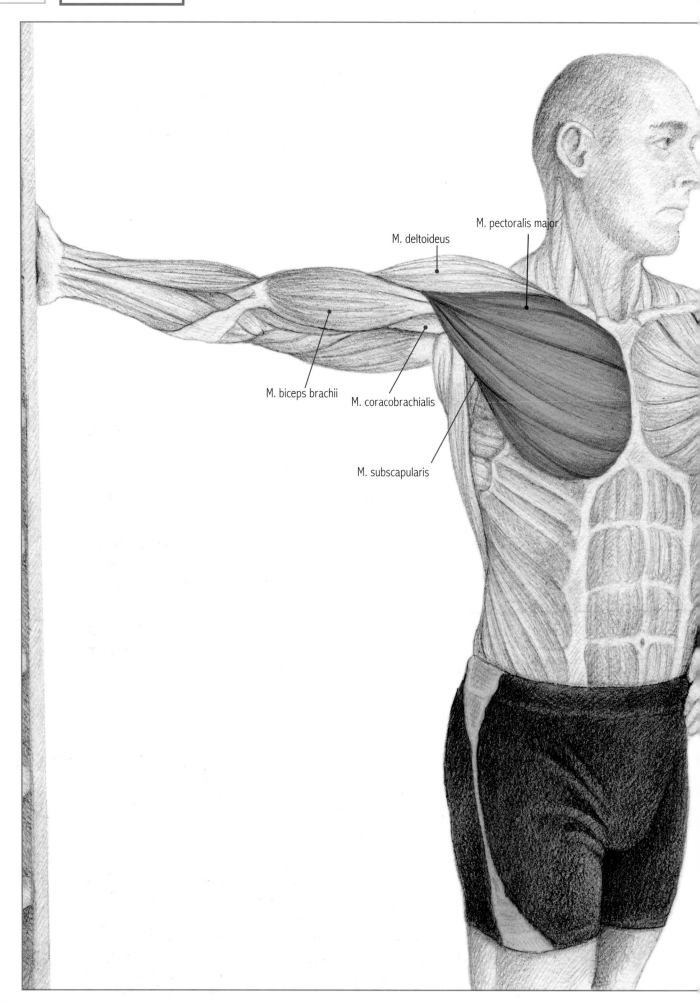

M. deltoideus

M. pectoralis major

M. biceps brachii

M. coracobrachialis

M. subscapularis

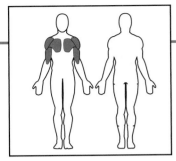

Muscles involved

Principal: Pectoralis major

Secondary: Anterior deltoid, biceps, coracobrachialis, subscapularis, pectoralis minor

Execution

While standing beside a wall or some other form of vertical support, raise the arm laterally (abduction) until shoulder height, with the palm of the hand facing forward so that it touches the support. The elbow remains slightly flexed. The arm and the pectoral region are then relaxed and the torso is rotated in the direction opposite to the raised arm.

Comments

This is a simple exercise, and it implies a whole series of muscles that are involved in the throwing movements in some sports (for example, baseball, javelin, etc.), most of the raquet sports (tennis, squash, etc.) as well as the hitting sports (boxing, martial arts).

If the tension on the arm makes it impossible to continue with the exercise, it can be kept slightly bent at the elbow.

On the other hand, although the difference is not great, if we elevate our arm a little above shoulder height, we will put a little more emphasis on the lower fibers of the pectoral muscle, whereas if we lower the hand, we target the upper fibers a little more. Curiously, this note seems to appear on the back of most stretching manuals, maybe due to the influence of strength-training.

The most common mistake is to put the tension in the pectoral area, as if you were attempting to push the wall, when in actuality, the feeling should be exactly the opposite. It is also not needed to extend the elbow completely since this is not a strecthing exercise for the arm.

Variation 1.2 .... With the elbow flexed

The position is similar, but the elbow is bent and the pushing is performed with the elbow rather than the hand. This stretch also involves the pectoral muscles, but not the flexors (for example, biceps, brachialis, etc.). Some manuals claim that what you achieve with this variant is more emphasis on the pectoralis minor, which is completely mistaken, since we know that the degree of flexion/extension of the elbow does not affect the degree of participation of this small muscle that runs from the ribs to the scapula, but not to the radius or ulna, or even to the humerus.

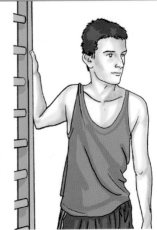

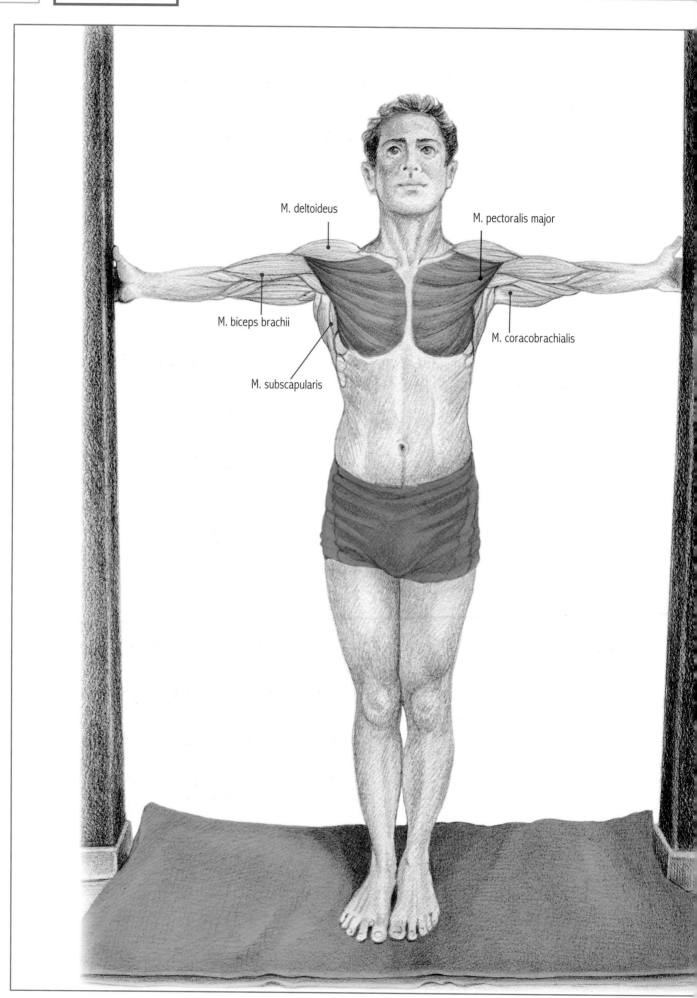

M. deltoideus

M. pectoralis major

M. biceps brachii

M. coracobrachialis

M. subscapularis

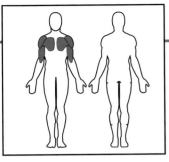

Muscles involved

Principal: Pectoralis major

Secondary: Anterior deltoid, biceps, coracobrachialis, subscapularis, pectoralis minor

Execution

From a standing position in front of a corner of the wall, raise your arms out in the shape of a cross (90° abduction) and lean forward, bringing the torso progressively closer to the corner.

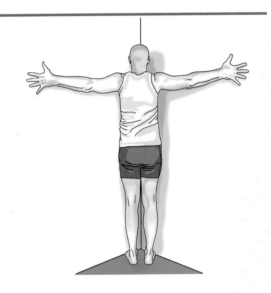

Comments

This simple stretching exercise involves both pectoralis majors, as well as the anterior portion of the deltoids and the arms.

As with the previous exercise, if the elbows are flexed and the push is done through the elbows, then the arm flexors will not undergo any stretching.

The most common mistake when performing this exercise is to remain with the feet stationary and letting the torso fall forward. The correct way to do this is to move forward slowly with small steps, bringing the entire body closer to the corner with the arms raised, otherwise you would be forcing the pectoralis muscles to contract in order to maintain the posture, when what we are aiming to do is relax them so they may be properly stretched.

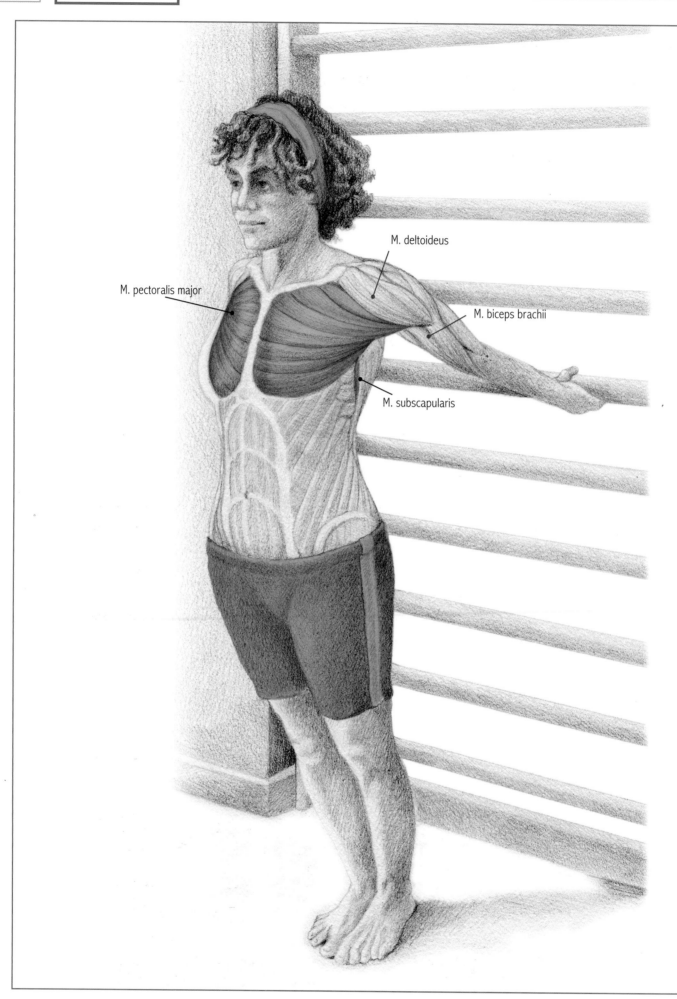

M. deltoideus

M. pectoralis major

M. biceps brachii

M. subscapularis

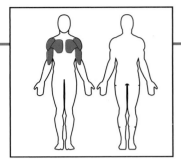

Muscles involved

Principal: Pectoralis major and subscapularis

Secondary: Anterior deltoid, biceps brachii, coracobrachialis

Execution

From a standing position, hold the bar behind you with a pronated grip (palms facing backward). Slowly let the body fall forward and downward.

Comments

The pronated grip allows us to avoid having the movement hindered by the elbow flexors, such as the biceps brachii. If you held the bar with a supine grip, then these muscles would also be stretched, something that must be done with special caution.

The position and the movement mean that the deltoids and other small muscles of the shoulder are also worked, particularly in the anterior region of the shoulder.

If the bar is placed too low, then the movement of the torso needs to be accompanied by a progressive bending of the knees, which allows for a greater extension of the arms.

Variation   3.2... With a partner

You can perform this stretching exercise with a partner who, standing back to back, holds either the bar or your hands. Then both partners simply allow their bodies to lean forward. Since with this variation there is a certain degree of unrest to maintain the commitment between stretching and balance, it is not as effective as the original variation described, performed individually.

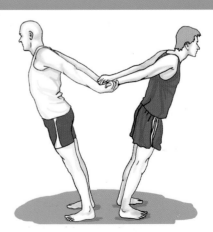

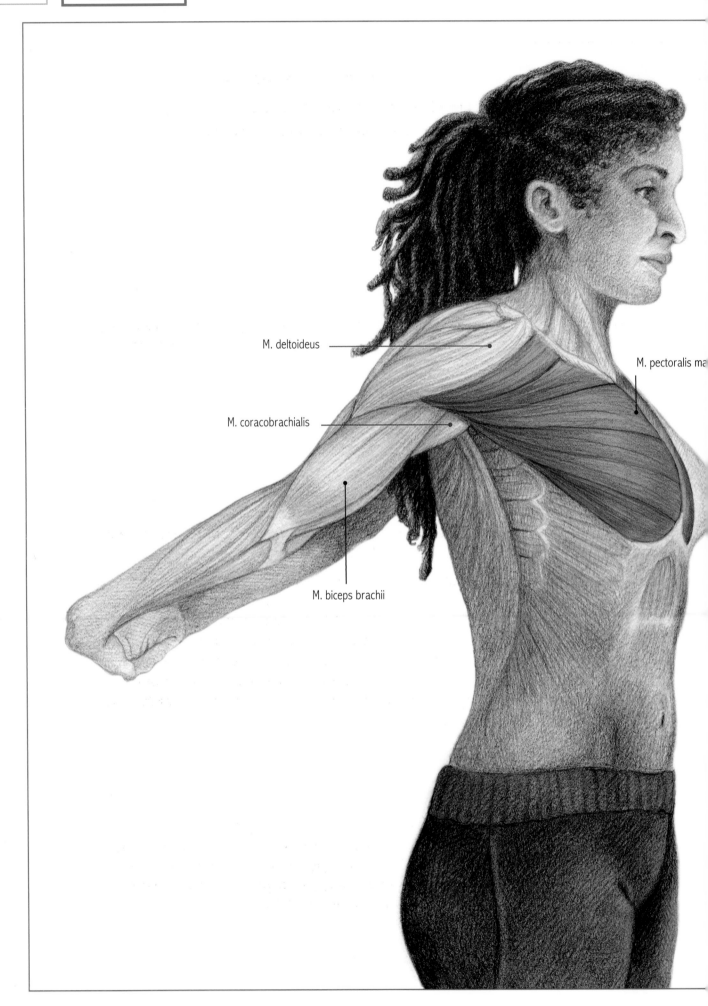

M. deltoideus

M. pectoralis ma[jor]

M. coracobrachialis

M. biceps brachii

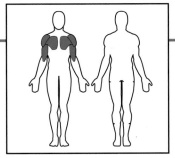

Muscles involved

Principal: Pectoralis major and subscapularis

Secondary: Anterior deltoid, biceps brachii, coracobrachialis

Execution

From a standing position, hold a wooden bar behind the body with a pronated grip (palms facing backward). Progressively elevate the arms in extension until you are able to feel the stretch in the pectoral region.

Comments

As with other exercises, using a pronated grip prevents the movement from being slowed by the elbow flexors, something that would happen more intensely if we held the bar with a supinated grip.

This exercise is similar to the previous one, but now it is the movement of our own muscles, rather than gravity, which creates the traction of the arms. Likewise, the position and the movement also make the shoulder work, especially the anterior portion of the deltoid. As with many other stretching exercises, the person performing this stretch must refrain from bouncing in an attempt to reach further limits. Unfortunately, without the help of a partner, it is hard to reach the limits necessary for improvement. The force of gravity and the tension to which the different muscles are exposed make this an exercise that may be useful for warming up or getting the stiffness out, but somewhat limited in terms of the results that can be obtained regarding increased range of motion.

 There are those who are unsure about whether they should stretch cold or after warming up. The answer is simple, in general terms warming up before stretching is safer from the point of view of injury prevention. The argument for stretching before warming up is more practical since it is our tendency to do so in every day life, but it lacks validity, given that physical exercises are outside of the scope of "everyday life," since progress requires us to go beyond our normal limits.

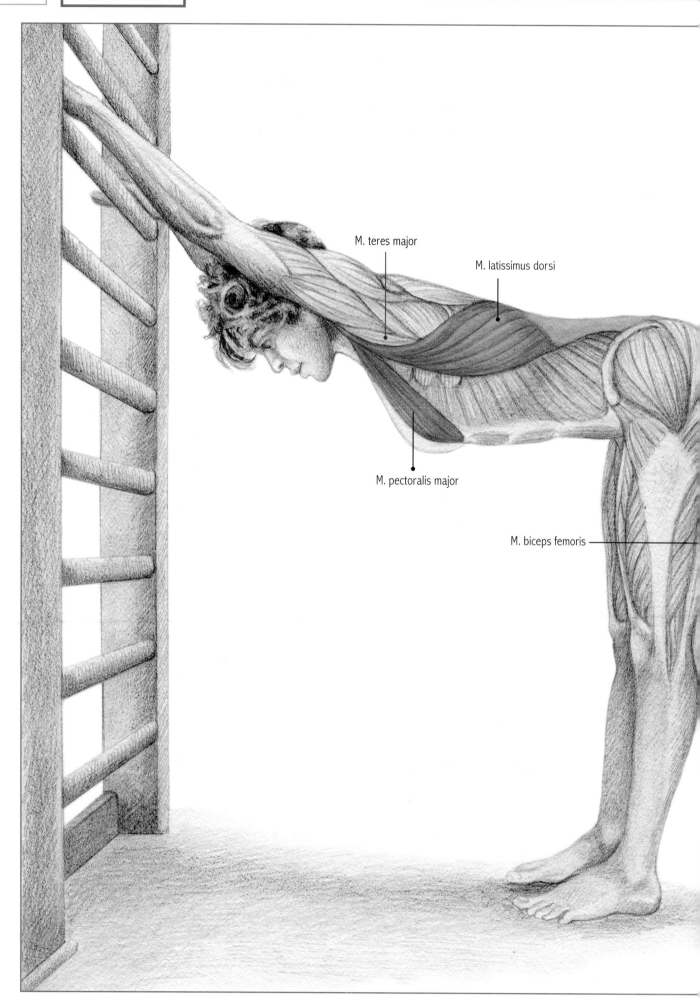

M. teres major

M. latissimus dorsi

M. pectoralis major

M. biceps femoris

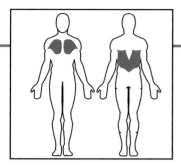

Muscles involved

Principal: Latissimus dorsi and pectoralis major

Secondary: Teres major (ischiotibial muscles)

Execution

Stand up and face a table or some other type of support that is approximately waist height. Place both hands on top of the table or support a little wider than shoulder-width apart, and then flex the torso down and progressively to the rear.

Comments

Although this exercise stretches different muscle groups, for the purpose of stretching the pectoral muscles, it is important to separate the arms well, otherwise, the latissimus dorsi and other muscles will be doing most of the work.

A slight variation, in which you lean on the table with the elbows flexed instead of with the hands, would not really affect the stretching of the pectoralis and latissimus dorsi, since both of these muscles insert into the upper arm and not the forearm. However, it may shift more of the stress toward the latissimus dorsi, as a result of having to keep the arms closer together.

Another variant, which is also effective and perhaps even slightly better, is to place yourself between two tables or supports of equal height, rest your arms on top of them and then perform the stretching exercise in the manner described above. This way, the latissimus dorsi receives less of the stretch and you are able to focus more of the effort upon the pectoralis major.

Variation   5.2... With a partner

If you happen to be outdoors and there is no support available, you may still be able to perform this stretching exercise with the help of a partner. Place your hands on each other's shoulders and perform the stretching exercise simultaneously. Ideally, your partner should have a wingspan similar to yours. Otherwise, if the difference is too great, then you will have to take turns, performing the exercise one after the other, with the resting partner just serving as support.

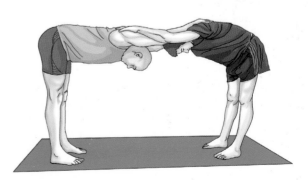

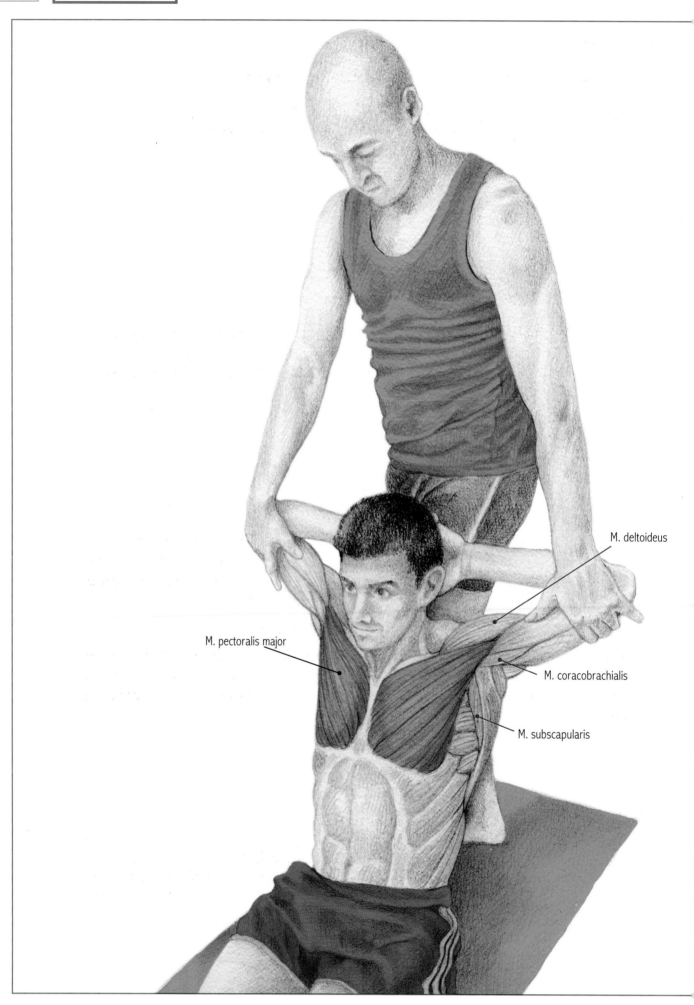

M. deltoideus

M. pectoralis major

M. coracobrachialis

M. subscapularis

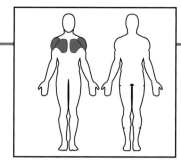

Muscles involved

Principal: Pectoralis major

Secondary: Anterior deltoid, subscapularis and coracobrachialis

Execution

Seated either on the ground or on a bench. Place your hands behind your head with the elbows at the height of the head. The partner will stand behind you, grab a hold of both of your hands and pull them upward and backward, at the same time, keeping your back still against his legs or the rear.

Comments

As with all stretching exercises for pairs, the force that the partner applies should be precise; other important things to note are watching the person and his reactions very closely, and estimating the limits of mobility with extreme caution. The correct way to assist in the performance of this exercise is to grab hold of the arms (not the elbows) around the lower tricep area.

In this case, the upper pecs are stretched slightly less than the lower pecs.

A very common mistake when assisting with the performance of this stretching exercise is when the partner digs the knee into the back and thus forces an arching of the back. Performing this exercise in front of a mirror has the added advantage wherein you can see each other´s faces and therefore communicate better.

 Can I injure myself while stretching? The answer is yes, particularly when you take a joint above and beyond its normal range of motion, or when the movement is performed compulsively. The lack of a warm-up, a poor diet or poor physical conditioning are other factors that may lead to injury during the performance of static stretches.

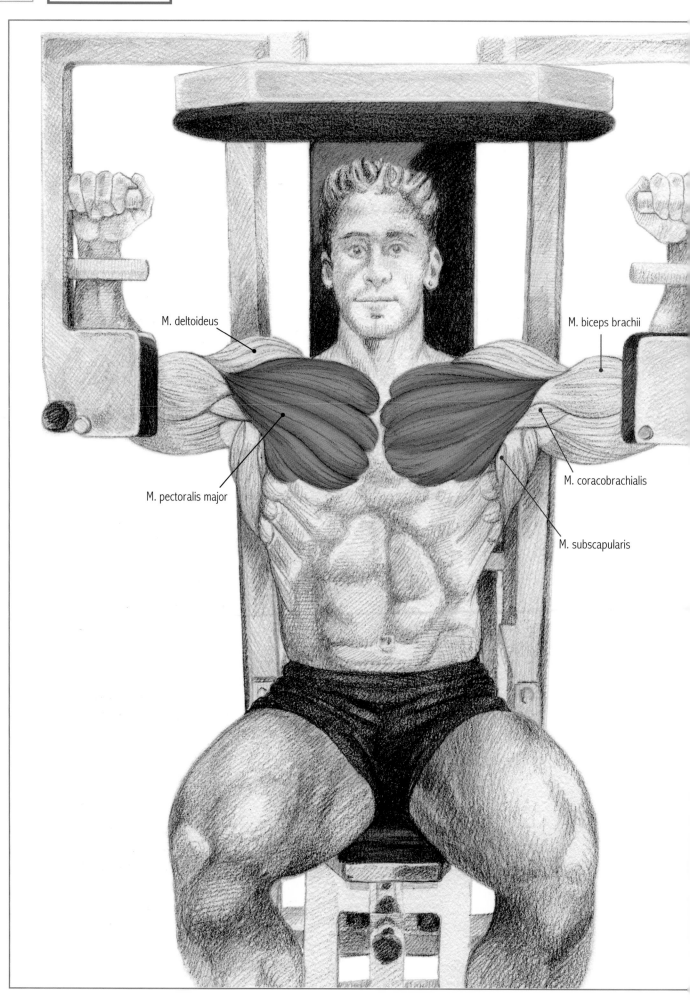

M. deltoideus

M. biceps brachii

M. pectoralis major

M. coracobrachialis

M. subscapularis

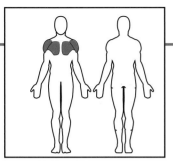

Muscles involved

Principal: Pectoralis major

Secondary: Anterior deltoids, subscapularis and coracobrachialis

Execution

Seated in a Peck-deck or "fly" machine (which is pretty much standard equipment in every gym) with the elboows resting on the pad, select an appropriate load and lift the weight with the legs (most machines will have this "load release" mechanism built in). Then get situated in position and proceed to slowly release the load with the legs to transfer it to the arms, passively, until it is the arms that are resisting all the weight. You do not finish by bringing the arms together, but rather by releasing the load once again with the legs.

Comments

This is a very simple, and above all, very effective stretching exercise, but it is imperative that the machine has that built-in load release mechanism (otherwise we are just begging to get injured). Furthermore, it is not necessary to put a lot of weight on the machine for this exercise to be effective, which is what people who are accustomed to using this equipment do as part of the strength building routine.

There are some variations of this machine in which the effort is done with the hands rather than with the elbows, and in that case, the elbow flexors also become involved. If this machine is not available, then a partner can help us attain the correct posture (see exercise 5).

The strength building machines, when properly chosen, can be of great help in stretching exercises. Some people do not use them because they consider them to be completely unrelated to their athletic discipline, but what is important is to train in an optimum way in order to achieve progress, and people´s prejudices about the value of one or another machine is really not important.

 INJURY — Pectoral tear: a rough movement during chest stretching may produce a muscle tear or a muscle strain. To avoid this, make sure the area is properly warmed up, and use slow, controlled, methodical movements along the complete range of motion for that joint. If you have already sustained an injury, then stop the physical activity, apply ice to the area immediately, and seek medical attention. If no major damage has been done, a few days of rest are usually enough to ensure a full recovery, whereas if a tear has occurred, it normally requires surgery to repair, followed by months of recovery.

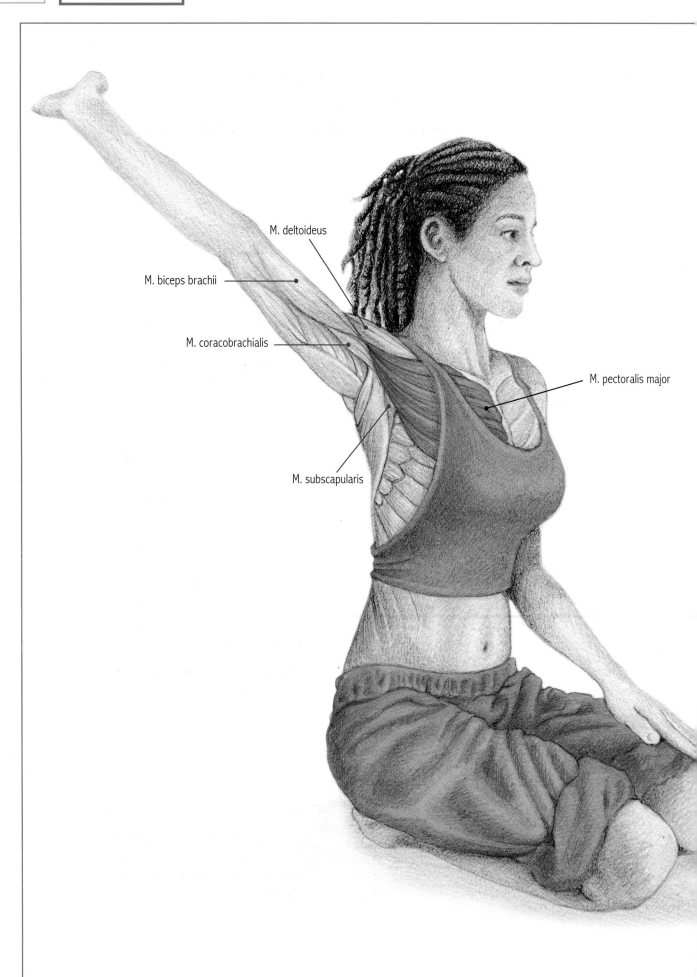

M. deltoideus

M. biceps brachii

M. coracobrachialis

M. pectoralis major

M. subscapularis

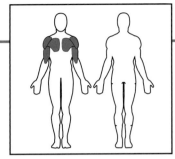

Muscles involved

Principal: Pectoralis major

Secondary: Anterior deltoids, biceps, coracobrachialis, subscapularis and pectoralis minor

Execution

A partner standing behind you will hold the torso with one hand and use the other hand to lift your arm backward and up.

Comments

The results obtained by performing this exercise are better if your training partner is strong enough to maintain the posture. If he isn't, then you should opt for such variants as the ones explained at the beginning of the chapter. Similarly, the training partner must attempt to keep the person stretching from twisting the torso, since doing so will nullify the stretching effect you are trying to achieve.

If the traction is on the forearm, thus forcing the subject to extend the elbow, this will also bring the elbow flexors into play. On the other hand, if the traction is from the elbow, the stretch will be much more isolated to the pectoral region.

 Do we need to include stretches as part of our regular training, or do we have to dedicate a specific training session just for stretching? The answer is, you should do both. A good way of thinking about it is this: Think of the specific stretching sessions as a means to improve flexibility and joint mobility, and think of the daily stretching as a way to maintain that and condition the body.

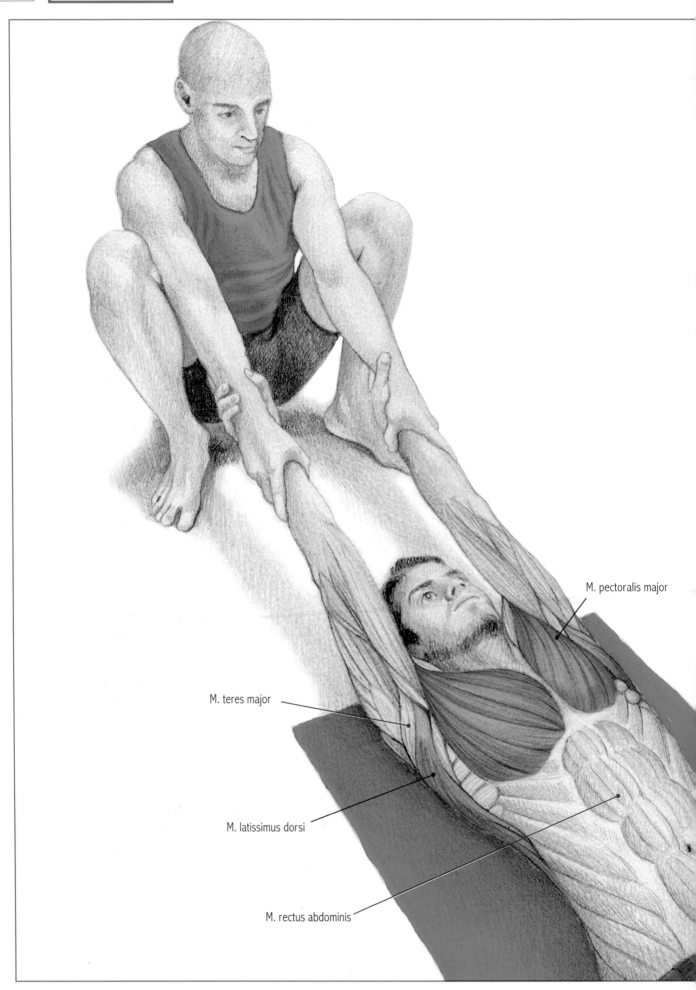

M. pectoralis major

M. teres major

M. latissimus dorsi

M. rectus abdominis

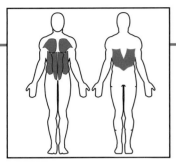

Muscles involved

Principal: Pectoralis major, latissimus dorsi

Secondary: Teres major, rectus abdominis

Execution

In a supine, decubitus position (lying flat on your back) with a partner sitting behind you, close to your head your partner will grab your arms and pull them toward him. You must allow yourself to be stretched and not maintain any tension in your body.

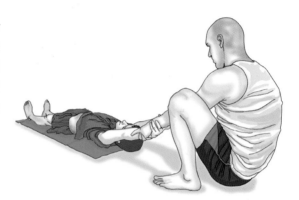

Comments

This exercise also involves the muscles of the back. With respect to the pectoral muscles, the area that is most stretched is the lower pectoral area. Due to the position of the shoulders and the type of traction, this exercise should be performed with caution by anyone who has problems with his / her shoulders.

On the other hand, while it is a good idea to choose a variety of exercises to stretch a particular muscle, this exercise is not one of the most effective for stretching the pectoral muscles, and there are better alternatives.

 Can you train to improve flexibility at any age? Yes, although you must keep in mind the degree of intensity of the stretches. However, unlike other physical qualities such as strength or endurance, stretching exercises can be initiated earlier in childhood, of course, in moderation and preferably as part of a game. The training sessions of boys and girls — who have not yet reached adolescence — in some of the highly competitive sports such as gymnastics, are an aberration that can sometimes lead to serious psychological consequences and almost always involves some physical consequences.

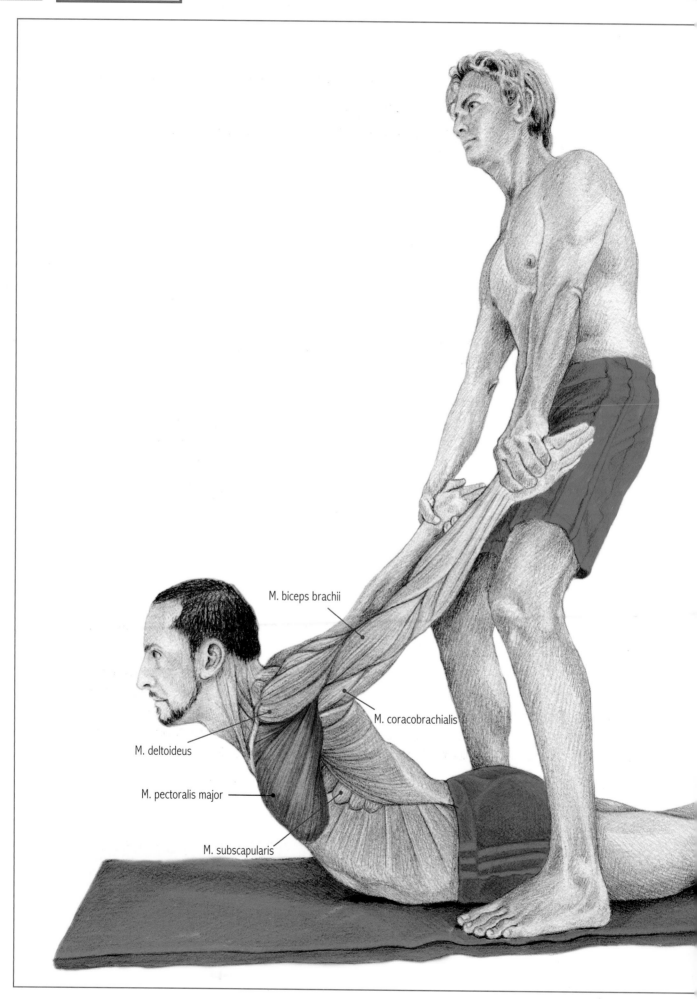

M. biceps brachii

M. coracobrachialis

M. deltoideus

M. pectoralis major

M. subscapularis

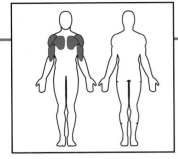

Muscles involved

Principal: Pectoralis major

Secondary: Anterior deltoids, biceps, coracobrachialis, subscapularis, pectoralis minor and serratus

Execution

From a decubitus prone position (lying face down) your partner pulls your arms up and back. The person being stretched may keep his or her arms extended or with the hands placed on the back of the head.

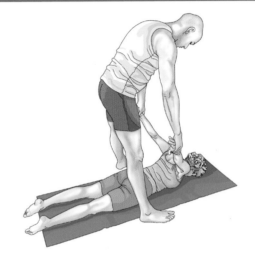

Comments

The pulling movement has to be very restrained. When the torso lifts off the floor, your partner should not pull any farther but hold that position instead.

The added difficulty for the person being stretched is knowing how to relax the pectoral region since the natural tendency is to want to place the arms in front of us to avoid falling and hitting the ground. This exercise should be avoided by those who suffer from recurrent dislocations of the shoulder joint. The person being stretched should also pay particular attention to his breathing, in an effort to keep it natural, since people tend to have difficulty maintaining their breathing during this exercise.

The relaxation and the descent following the stretch should also be gentle and slow.

 What are the keys to training with a partner? Three in particular:

1. Knowing exactly which exercise is going to be performed.

2. Always be slow and methodical when helping your partner stretch.

3. Have an established signal between you and your partner in order to stop when you have reached the limit.

Descriptive anatomy of the back muscles:
a biomechanical introduction to the principal muscles involved

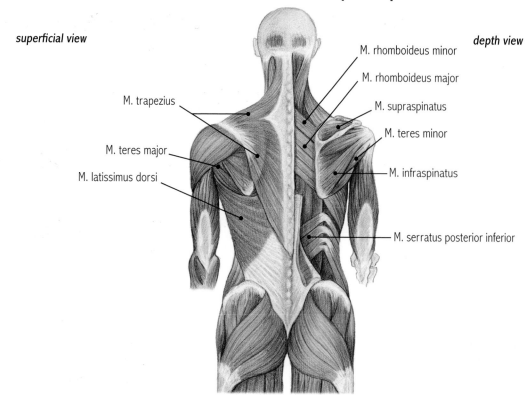

superficial view

depth view

M. trapezius

M. teres major

M. latissimus dorsi

M. rhomboideus minor

M. rhomboideus major

M. supraspinatus

M. teres minor

M. infraspinatus

M. serratus posterior inferior

With insertion into the humerus

Latissimus dorsi (posterior, superficial)

Origin: Thoracic vertebrae (spinous processes of T7 through T12), thoracolumbar fascia and iliac crest (posterior third), ribs (costal segment of the 10th to 12th ribs), and almost always also in the scapula (inferior angle)

Insertion: Humerus (greater tubercle and crest)

Principal functions: Adduction of the arm when it is raised, internal rotation (put into doubt by some expert); also assists in the extension of the humerus and bringing the scapula in toward the spinal column

Teres minor (posterior, deep)

Origin: Scapula (lateral border)

Insertion: Humerus (lesser tubercle and crest)

Principal functions: Weak lateral rotation of the arm; assists in the adduction of the arm

Teres major (posterior, superficial)

Origin: Scapula (lateral inferior border)

Insertion: Humerus (lesser tubercle or subtrochanter)

Principal functions: Retroversion, adduction and weak internal rotation of the arm

Infraspinatus (posterior, deep)

Origin: Scapula (infraspinous fossa and spine of the scapula)

Insertion: Humerus (medial aspect of greater tubercle)

Principal functions: Lateral rotation of the arm and stabilizes the shoulder joint capsule

Brief comment: The powerful and spectacular latissimus dorsi is underutilized in a sedentary lifestyle, but it is very important in a large number of sporting activities. Unfortunately, just like other muscles of the region, it is often the target of pain caused by contractures and rigidity. Furthermore, since it is an area that is difficult to reach on our own bodies, many people turn to massages in their search for relief. But stretches help to prevent and assist in the improvement of all kinds of back ailments.

omboid major (posterior, deep)

gin: Thoracic vertebrae (spinous processes of T1-T4)

ertion: Scapula (medial border)

ncipal functions: Adduction of the scapula; retraction of the sca-
a toward the spinal column and maintaining it there; elevation of the
pula

Rhomboid minor (posterior, deep)

Origin: Cervical vertebrae (spinous processes of C7 and C8)

Insertion: Scapula (internal border)

Principal functions: Retraction of the scapula toward the spinal column and maintaining it there

apezius (posterior, superficial)

"SHOULDERS"

Levator scapulae (posterior-superior, medium)

See "SHOULDERS"

rratus minor posterior and inferior (posterior-inferior, deep)

"ABDOMEN"

Illiocostals (posterior, deep)

See "ABDOMEN" (and lumbars)

Brief comment: The torso is the pillar of the body where all of the other body parts find support in order to perform their respective functions, whether directly or indirectly. It is not possible to individually stretch the majority of the muscles of the back, but it does do part of the work in various exercises aimed for other body parts. This is one of the reasons why diversifying the exercises one performs is important in muscle stretching.

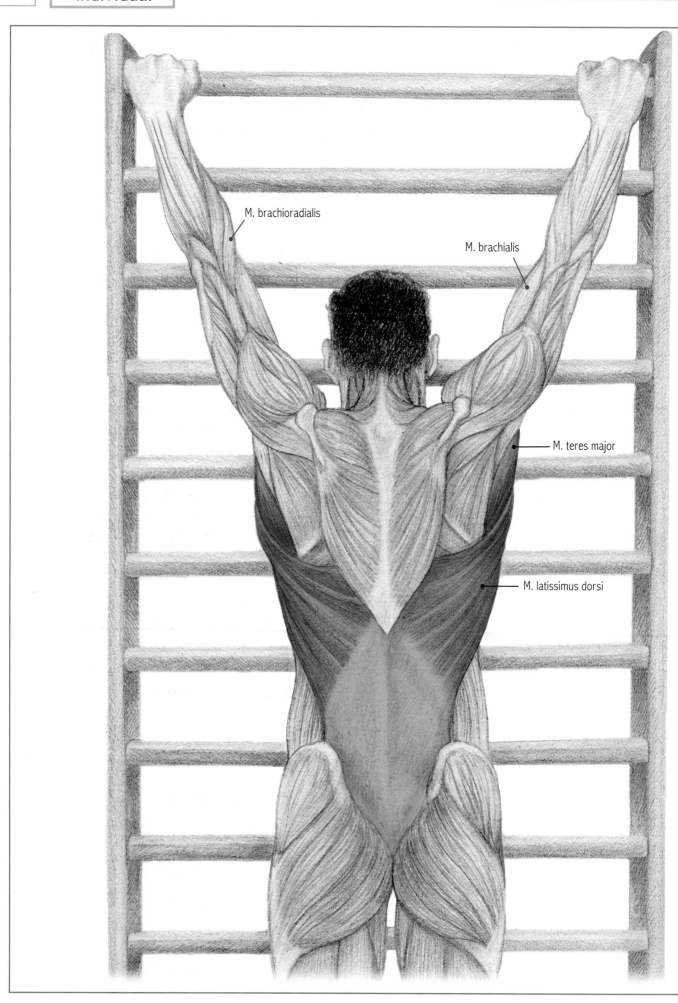

M. brachioradialis

M. brachialis

M. teres major

M. latissimus dorsi

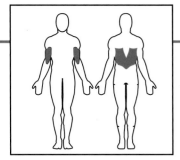

Muscles involved

Principal: Latissimus dorsi, teres major

Secondary: Biceps, brachialis, brachioradialis, pectorals

Execution

Grab a bar with a pronated grip (palms facing forward) and let yourself hang from it without letting your feet touch the floor; hold this position without tension.

Comments

This is a simple exercise. The farther apart your hands are, the more emphasis that will be placed on the lateral portions of the back. On the other hand, with a supinated grip, you will place more emphasis on the biceps.

Hanging from a bar is an excellent exercise for relaxing various structures along the length of the vertebral column. We should realize that most of the time, the back is under a significant amount of tension and that this exercise pulls the entire structure with just the help of gravity. Among those who derive the greatest benefit are people with deviations of the spinal column (for example, hyperlordosis, hyperkyphosis and especially scoliosis). In the case of hyperlordosis, it is also important to flex the waist and knees (rounding up) to further stretch the lumbar region.

Some people choose to use a lumbar belt (like the ones used in weightlifting) to add some extra weight. This must be done with caution since too much weight can damage the column. Remember that it is designed to support a lot of weight vertically, not to tolerate significant pulling forces.

From the hanging position, it is permissibe to perform slight rotations of the torso, but never to the point where the limits of motion are reached because this could injure the small rotator muscles of the spine.

| Variation | 1.2... On a pull-down machine |

The exercise can be performed in an almost identical way by holding on to the bar of the lat pulldown machine. Beginners, or those with a problem or a weakness in their grip, may find this to be a good alternative although it is recommended that you select a weight that is somewhat challenging.

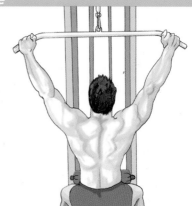

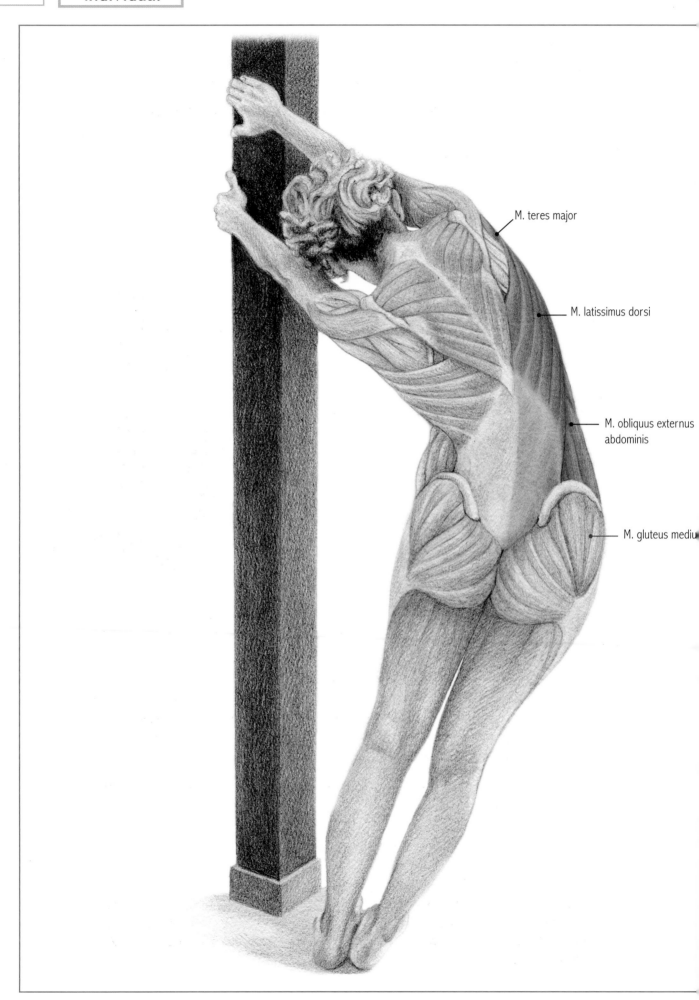

M. teres major

M. latissimus dorsi

M. obliquus externus abdominis

M. gluteus mediu

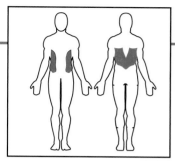

Muscles involved

Principal: Latissimus dorsi, teres major, abdominal obliques, quadratus lumborum

Secondary: Gluteus medius, tensor fascia lata

Execution

Stand next to a vertical bar and position your feet close to the bar. Grab the bar above your head and let your body fall to the opposite side. Both hands hold on to the bar on the same side, with palms facing forward.

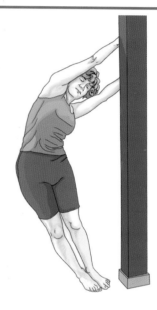

Comments

Although the tension will only be placed on the side opposite the bar, the opposite hand must still hold on to the bar in order to regulate how much the body falls.

The muscle areas that are worked are very similar to those in exercise 1, but here you are able to get a greater back stretch, and other areas of the back are also involved. When this exercise is done correctly, you can easily feel how the entire side of the torso is being stretched. If we want to emphasize the muscles of the hip a little more (the gluteus medius and the tensor fascia lata) cross the leg that is farther away from the bar behind the leg that is closer to the bar.

A common mistake is the tendency to rotate the torso so that you are facing the bar, but to do this exercise correctly, the body must remain sideways.

 Before stretching any muscle, you should think about it and visualize it and remember where it originates and where it inserts. Once we have thought about this, then we can proceed with the stretching. It is of no use to adopt a stretching posture if we have not even thought about the muscles we are going to be stretching.

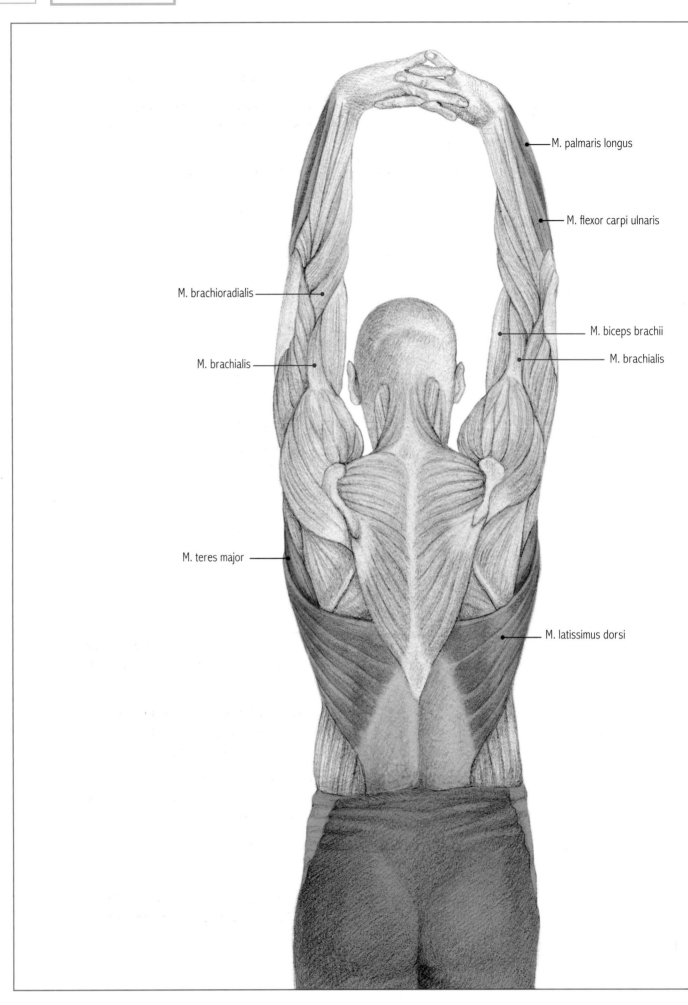

M. palmaris longus

M. flexor carpi ulnaris

M. brachioradialis

M. biceps brachii

M. brachialis

M. brachialis

M. teres major

M. latissimus dorsi

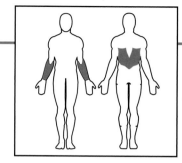

Muscles involved

Principal: Latissimus dorsi, teres major, finger flexors (flexor digitorum superficialis and profundus and flexor hallucis longus), flexor carpi ulnaris, long and short palmar muscles

Secondary: Biceps, brachialis, brachioradialis, pectorals

Execution

Standing up, preferably in front of a mirror, raise your arms above your head, with fingers interlaced and palms facing upward. Stretch as if reaching for the ceiling.

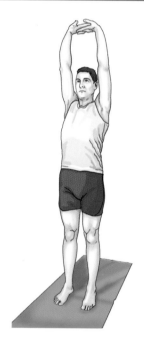

Comments

This exercise is very similar to the two previous ones in terms of the area of the back that is being stretched, but the intensity is somewhat less. Additionally, this exercise also involves the flexors of the hand.

Unlike the two previous exercises, this is an exercise that can be performed by people of advanced age and those with physical disabilities (depending on the type and degree of the disability). The latter two groups of people can omit interlacing the fingers if it presents a problem.

While performing this exercise, some people tend to stand on the tips of their toes as they try to stretch even more parts of the body. Although in principle this is not harmful, it may prevent the person from concentrating and compromise his or her stability. We should focus on stretching the muscle we want to stretch, without complicating matters unnecessarily.

 In flexibility training, mirrors provide a reference and serve as an aid to help us verify whether our body position is appropriate. They should never be used to criticize the image that we project on them; we are not judging our appearance but rather our posture.

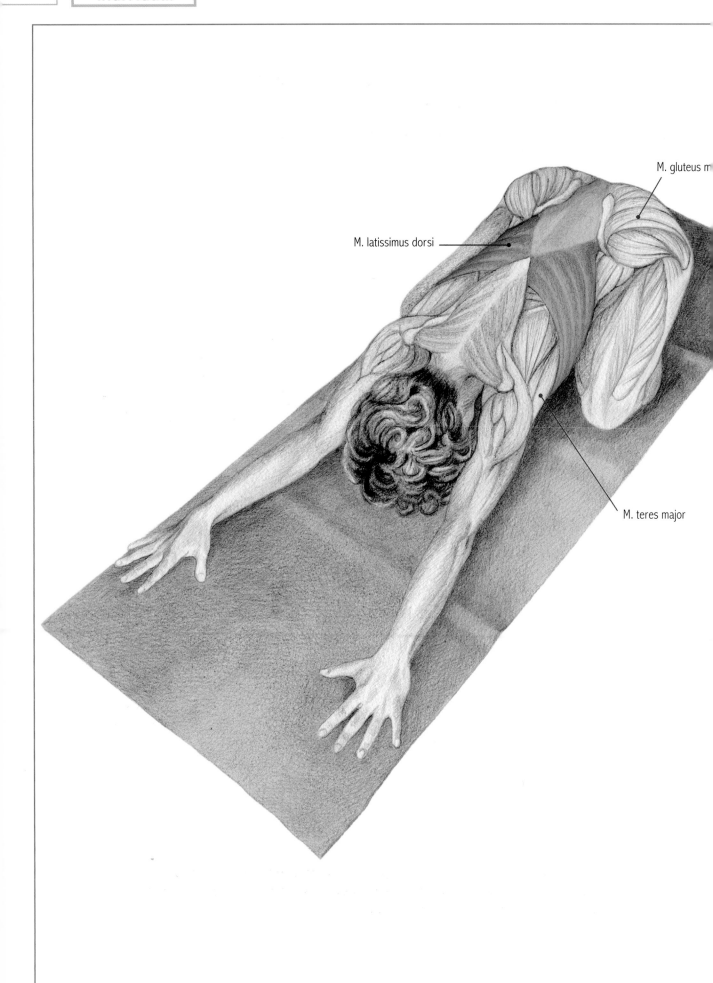

M. gluteus m

M. latissimus dorsi

M. teres major

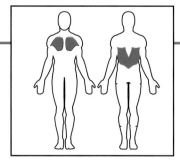

Muscles involved

Principal: Latissimus dorsi, pectoralis major

Secondary: Teres major, gluteus maximus

Execution

With your knees on the ground (preferably on top of a padded mat), flex the torso and rest your hands on the ground in front of you, beyond your head. Lower your waist downward and back, maintaining your elbows straight and your hands fixed on the ground at the same time that you press your torso downward toward the floor.

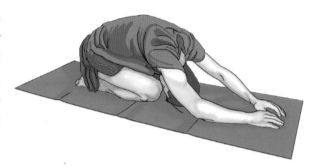

Comments

The name that we have given to this exercise is very indicative of the posture that needs to be adopted, but we should not forget about the tension that needs to be produced in the dorsal area during the traction of the torso. The hands should not be placed too far apart unless we want to involve the pectorals too much. In the finishing position, the chest rests on top of the thighs and the shoulders are pressed lightly against the ground, although it may also be performed without this support. This exercise can also be performed in a similar way by placing the hands on top of a support (see exercise 5).

 Flexibility is very much related to two other physical and mental disciplines: relaxation and corporal expression. For example, one session of flexibility training performed in a warm, relaxing atmosphere is not only more gratifying, it is also much more effective.

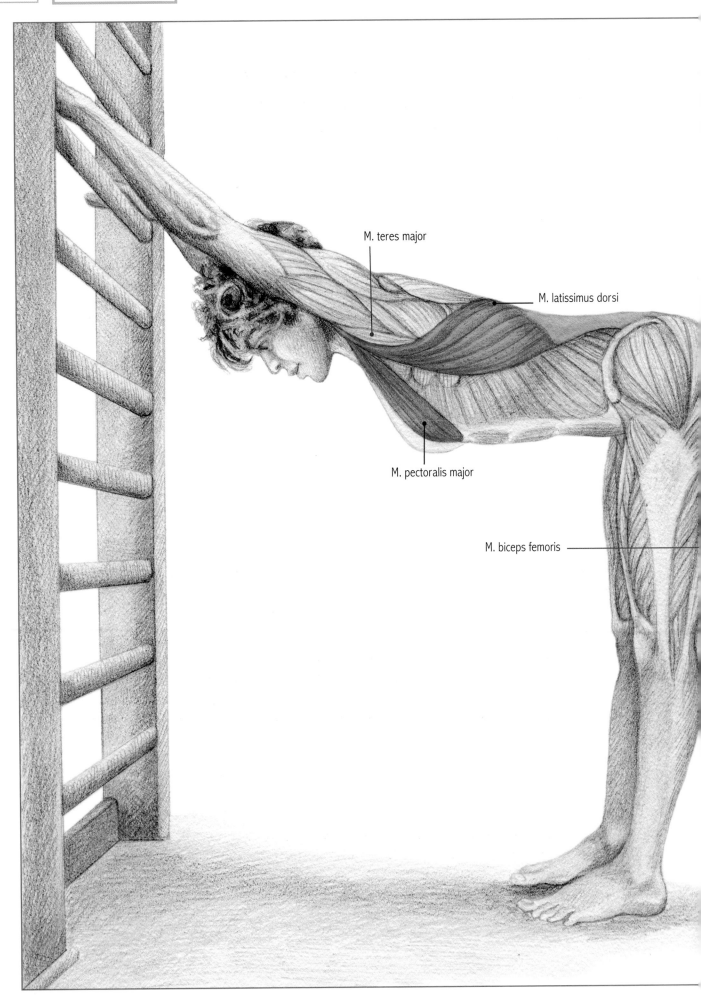

M. teres major

M. latissimus dorsi

M. pectoralis major

M. biceps femoris

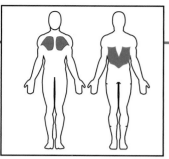

Muscles involved

Principal: Latissimus dorsi, pectoralis major

Secondary: Teres major, (ischiotibialis)

Execution

Standing up and facing a support that is higher than your waist, flex the torso and rest the hands above it, preferably with the arms externally rotated (supporting the fists, with the pinky finger on the surface). Keeping the arms immobile, lower the torso even farther until you can feel the stretch in the target area.

Comments

The latissimus dorsi muscle gets even more of a stretch if you perform this movement with a slight external rotation of the arms. Therefore, it may be more comfortable to perform this exercise while holding on to vertical bars rather than over a table or another flat surface. This will also allow your body to hang back a little bit more, so that we are farther from our support and there is a little extra added to the stretching of the torso. If there is no such support available, then an alternative is to perform this exercise on the ground (see exercise 4).

During this exercise, the pectoral muscles and others will inevitably also be stretched, but there is a small variation that increases the stretch of the dorsal muscles. To do this, hold on with only one arm and, as you pull backwards and down, slightly twist the pelvis and the spine away from the outstretched arm, thereby arching the torso laterally. This is more easily achieved by moving back the foot on the side that is being stretched.

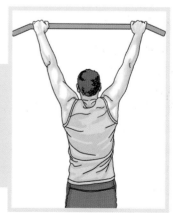

 In those exercises in which you hold onto a fixed support, there is a tendency to tense the muscles that you shouldn't be tensing. In a grip, it is the forearm and the small muscles of the hand that allow us to hold on. The area that we are going to stretch needs to be relaxed. This requires patience and learning, but it needs to be done this way in order to achieve better results.

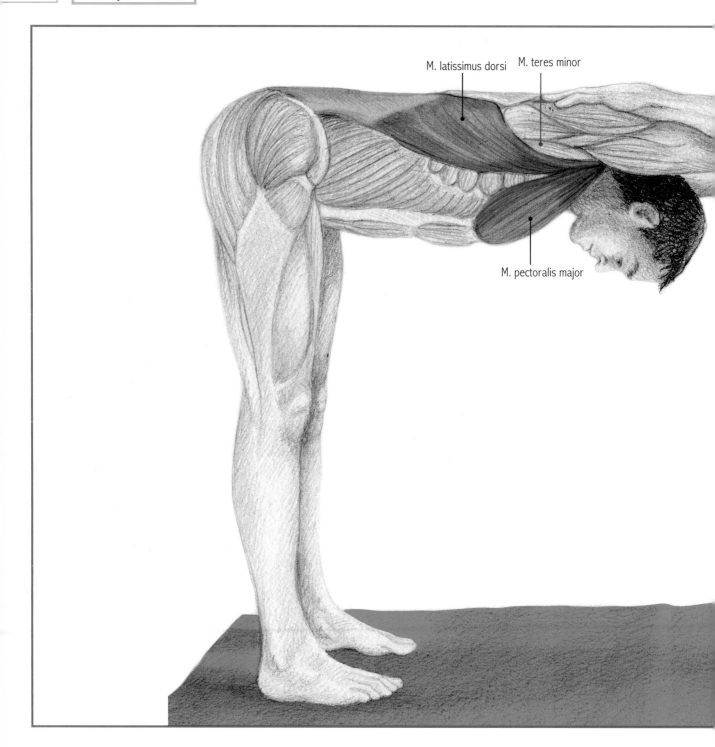

M. latissimus dorsi   M. teres minor

M. pectoralis major

Comments

With this exercise, the results are better if both partners are of a similar height and weight. If there is too much of a height difference, it is advisable to have the shorter member of the pair stand on a step. If the differences in weight are also significant, it would be better to perform a different exercise instead, such as holding on to a bar, for example (see exercise 5).

The pull backwards should not be too strong because, otherwise, the partner will also have to exert himself to compensate and it will become a rivalry that will prevent the necessary relaxation to achieve a good outcome. Instead of this, more pressure should be applied downward.

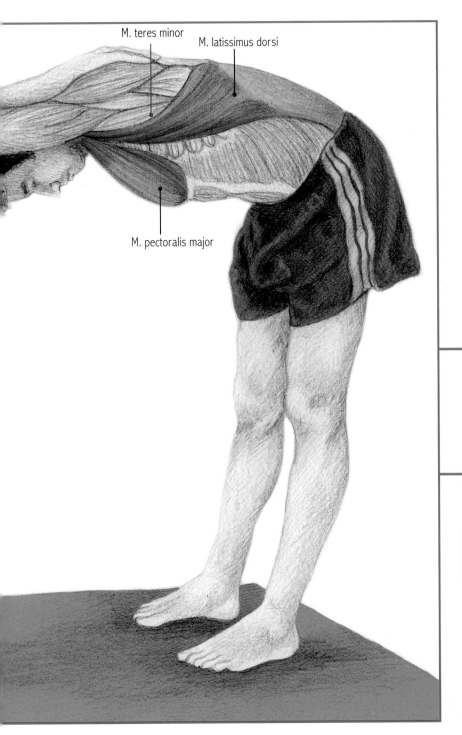

M. teres minor

M. latissimus dorsi

M. pectoralis major

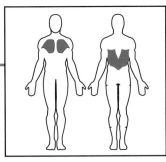

Muscles involved

Principal: Latissimus dorsi, pectoralis major

Secondary: Teres major

Execution

Standing up and facing your partner, hold each other by interlocking your arms, flex ninety degrees at the waist and pull backwards and down at the same time.

 Training with a person of the same or opposite sex should not pose any difficulty. It makes no difference. The only prerequisite is to treat the other person with respect.

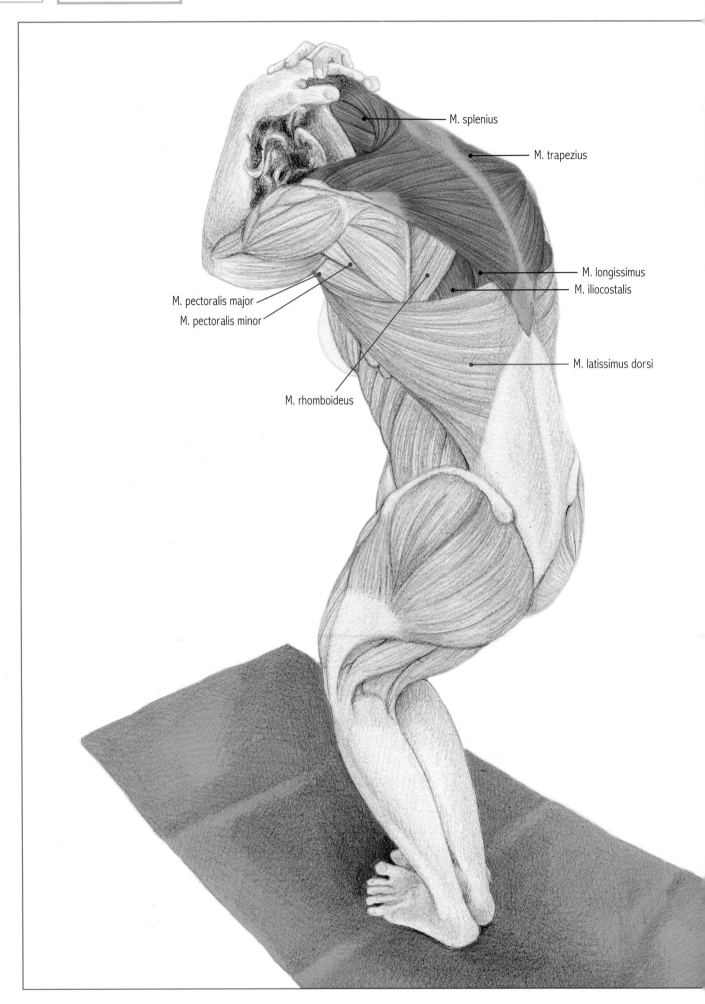

M. splenius

M. trapezius

M. longissimus

M. iliocostalis

M. pectoralis major

M. pectoralis minor

M. latissimus dorsi

M. rhomboideus

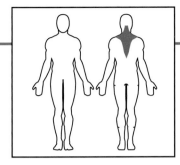

Muscles involved

Principal: Dorsalis longus, iliocostals, transversospinal and semispinalis, multifidus, trapezius, semispinal and splenius muscles

Secondary: Rectus capitis posterior major and minor, obliquus capitis inferior and superior, quadratum laborum

Execution

From a standing position, place your hands on the back of your head and pull gently downward at the same time that we arch our entire body in a light flexion of the torso, waist, and knees.

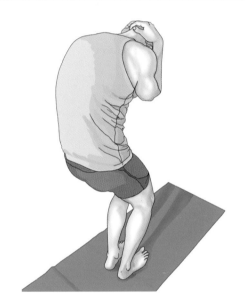

Comments

The feeling that must be experienced when performing this exercise is feeling the stretch and lengthening of all the muscles that surround the vertebral column down the back, as if forming an arch where we separate the two ends. If you have a difficult time maintaining your balance, you may rest one of the glutes against the wall for some added support.

Some common mistakes when performing this exercise are pulling too hard and executing the movement too rapidly. If you develop a headache or become dizzy with this type of exercise, then it is better to avoid this type of exercise where you are pulling on the head; it is possible that you may derive enough benefit from flexibility and mobility training using exercises where you can maintain an adequate stretching posture without the added force of the hands.

 At times, we treat the various body areas as if they were independent of each other, although this may be helpful when it comes to studying the muscle groups, explaining them or understanding them. When one is stretching, he or she needs to remember the muscle chains and the various relationships among the different areas of the body.

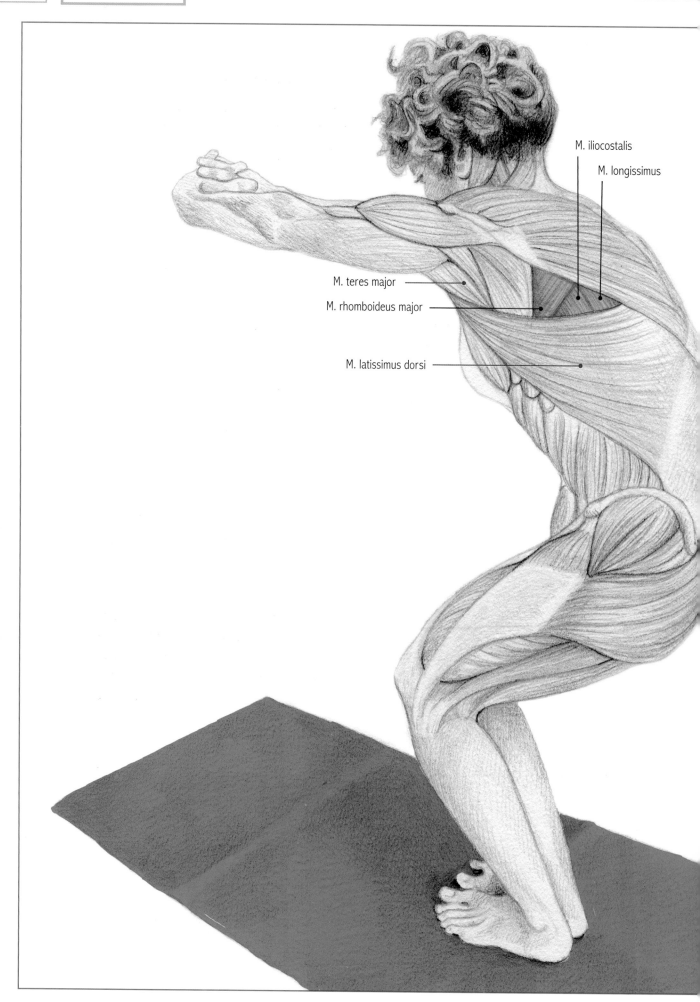

M. iliocostalis

M. longissimus

M. teres major

M. rhomboideus major

M. latissimus dorsi

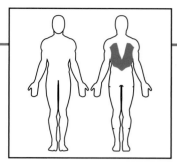

Muscles involved

Principal: Dorsalis longus, iliocostals, transversospinal and semispinalis, multifidus, trapezius, semispinal and rhombus major and minor

Secondary: Latissimus dorsi, teres major (quadratum laborum)

Execution

While standing, extend the arms forward with the fingers interlaced and the palms facing outward and forward. Curve your back at the same time that you "push" forward with the palms of your hands.

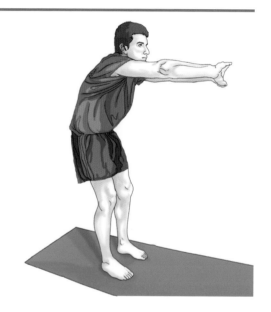

Comments

The posture for this exercise may be similar to the one before (see exercise 7) and in this way achieves a stretch of the autochthonous muscles of the spine. But on this particular occasion, we want the emphasis to be on the rhomboids, which are primarily tasked with bringing the scapulae in toward the spine. Thus, the stretching movement is precisely the opposite. We must try to lift the scapulae to the outside and forward (the arms extended forward are just an aid for execution, since it could be performed with the elbows flexed).

The knees and waist must remain slightly flexed to help maintain posture.

Certain common mistakes result from adopting the wrong position, just as some people are set on extending the arms forward, and upon noting the stretch in the arms, they mistakenly believe that they are performing the exercise correctly. Quite the contrary, the feeling of being stretched must come from the region of the upper back.

 Mobilize the scapulae and stretch the small muscles of the area (such as the rhomboids). This is a prophylactic treatment against back contractures.)

3

Descriptive anatomy of the muscles of the neck and shoulders: a biomechanical introduction to the principal muscles involved

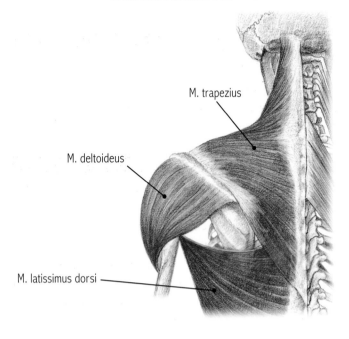

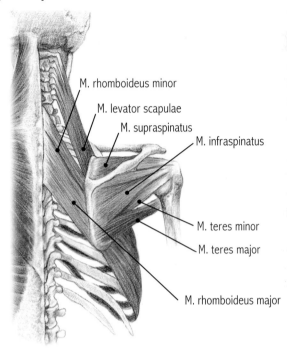

M. trapezius

M. deltoideus

M. latissimus dorsi

M. rhomboideus minor

M. levator scapulae

M. supraspinatus

M. infraspinatus

M. teres minor

M. teres major

M. rhomboideus major

Muscles that insert into the humerus

Deltoid: (lateral and superficial)

Origin: Clavicle, lateral one third of its anterior portion = haz 1 and 2; Acromium, medial portion = haz 3; Scapula, in the inferior border of its spine, its posterior/spinal portion = haz 4, 5, 6, and 7

Insertion: Humerus (deltoid or "in V" tuberosity)

Principal functions: Powerful abduction of the arm from 0 to 90° (between 0 and 30° by the acromion and then the rest is added), anteversion and internal rotation of the clavicle, retroversion and external rotation of the spine.

Coracobrachialis: (anterior and middle)

Origin: Scapula (coracoid process)

Insertion: Humerus (medial surface)

Principal functions: Anteversion of the arm and assists in maintaining the head of the humerus in the glenoid fossa; assists secondarily in adduction of the arm

Supraspinatus (superior, lateral and deep)

Origin: Supraspinous fossa

Insertion: Humerus (upper aspect of the greater tubercle)

Principal functions: Abduction of the arm, keeping the head of the humerus inside of the glenoid fossa

Teres minor (posterior and deep)

See "DORSAL"

Infraspinatus (posterior and deep)

See "DORSAL"

Subscapularis (anterior and deep)

See "PECTORAL"

Teres major

See "DORSAL"

Brief comments: As it is well known, the hypertonic dorsal and pectoral muscles can cause dislocations; the biceps, supraspinatus, suprascapularis, infraspinatus, teres minor and others inhibit and delay the dislocation. In fact, the freedom in the range of motion the shoulder joint enjoys also predisposes it to dislocation. And while here we may consider the deltoids and adjacent muscles as being a group of muscles specific for this joint, there are actually several different muscle groups affecting the joint. Any person predisposed to suffering a shoulder dislocation should consult with his or her physician before initiating any of the stretching exercises.

Muscles that do not insert into the humerus

apezius (posterior and superficial)

gin: Head (descending/superior part in the posterior midline, ernal occipital protuberance and ligament); cervical and thoracic tebrae (C7-T3) in the spinous processes and supraspinal ligament; racic vertebrae (ascending/inferior portion) T2 or T3 through T12

ertion: Clavicle (descending/superior portion in the lateral third; nsverse/medial in the acromial process and acromium; Scapula cending/inferior portion in the triangular portion or adjacent to it)

ncipal functions: Elevation of the shoulder and hyperlordosis h rotation toward opposite side and lateral rotation toward the side its head (superior portion; scapular adduction; approximation of shoulders toward the rear (middle portion); scapular depression; placement of the shoulder down and inward (inferior portion); bilizer of the scapula and scapular waist; abduction of the humerus

ernocleidomastoid (anterior superior)

igin: Sternum (manubrium or tendinous head) and clavicle (internal rd, the muscle head)

ertion: Head (mastoid and superior nuchal line)

ncipal functions: Flexion of head and neck: turning head to posite side, tilting head to ipsilateral side

Levator scapulae

Origin: Cervical vertebrae (transverse processes of the first four)

Insertion: Scapula (superior angle)

Principal functions: Elevation and adduction of the scapula, medially rotates inferior angle

OTHERS

Posterior rectus major: Axis to occipital. Extension of the head, contributes to lateral inclination and ipsilateral rotation

Posterior rectus minor: Atlas to occipital. Extension of the head, contributes to lateral inclination

Major oblique: Axis to atlas. Backward movement and extension of the atlas over the axis, contributes to lateral inclination and ipsilateral rotation

Minor oblique: Atlas to occipital. Extension of the head, contributes to lateral inclination and contralateral rotation

Scalene: Vertebrae to ribs. Inclination and homolateral rotation

Interspinosus: Between cervical spinous processes. Extension of the column

Serratus anterior: (anterior, deep)
See "PECTORAL"

Pectoralis minor: (anterior, deep)
See "PECTORAL"

Rhomboid major: (posterior, deep)
See "DORSAL"

Rhomboid minor: (posterior, deep)
See "DORSAL"

Brief comments: Along with the back, the neck is one of the areas that suffer the greatest tension and pain due to our lifestyle. If you ask any massage therapist, they will confirm this.

Stretching the muscles of the neck is simple, but doing it carefully is an absolute must. The neck exercises must not be taken to the extremes of mobility, and they also cannot be prolonged like those for other areas. Too much stretching can cause a headache. Furthermore, although in our everyday routines it may not seem like much to us, the head is actually very heavy (it weighs approximately 5 kg) and it is located above delicate joint structures. The mass of the head, falling with gravity, can result in injury if it is not done in a controlled fashion.

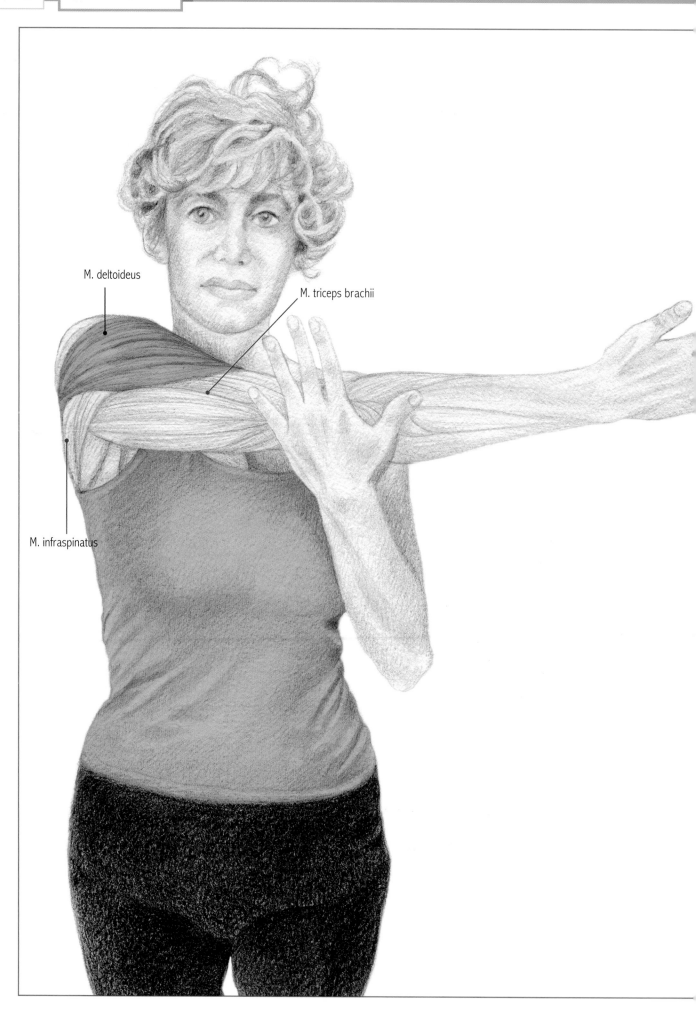

M. deltoideus

M. triceps brachii

M. infraspinatus

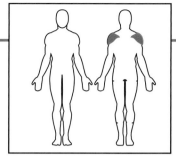

Muscles involved

Principal: Rear deltoids

Secondary: Rhomboids, triceps, infraspinatus, teres minor, teres major

Execution

Either standing up or sitting down, in front of a mirror, raise the arm in front by flexing the shoulder, and with the opposite hand press the elbow toward the chest and back.

Comments

As it is well known, the deltoid can produce movement in many different directions, subdivided into at least 3 (according to each ot its heads) or even into seven different subcategories (according to one classification study.) The exercise pictured here centers on the rear motions, although it also stretches the adjacent muscles, particularly the rhomboids.

If the stretching is done horizontally, as the image shows, the entire back region of the deltoid is stretched. If it is done raising the arm toward the face, the stress is shifted slightly toward the lower fibers of the rear deltoid as well as the teres minor. Doing the inverse, shifts the emphasis toward the upper rear fibers and the supraspinatus. In any case, the pressure exerted by the non-stretched arm must be significant, and the risk of injury is not high if it is performed with a controlled movement (but particular caution, as always, applies to people who have recurrent dislocation problems).

 The concept of the "shoulders" is a little bit vague. It would be more appropriate to talk of a scapulo-humeral joint, or an acromio-clavicular or scapulo-thoracic joint. But in general, the term refers to the upper joint of the arm and adjacent structures.

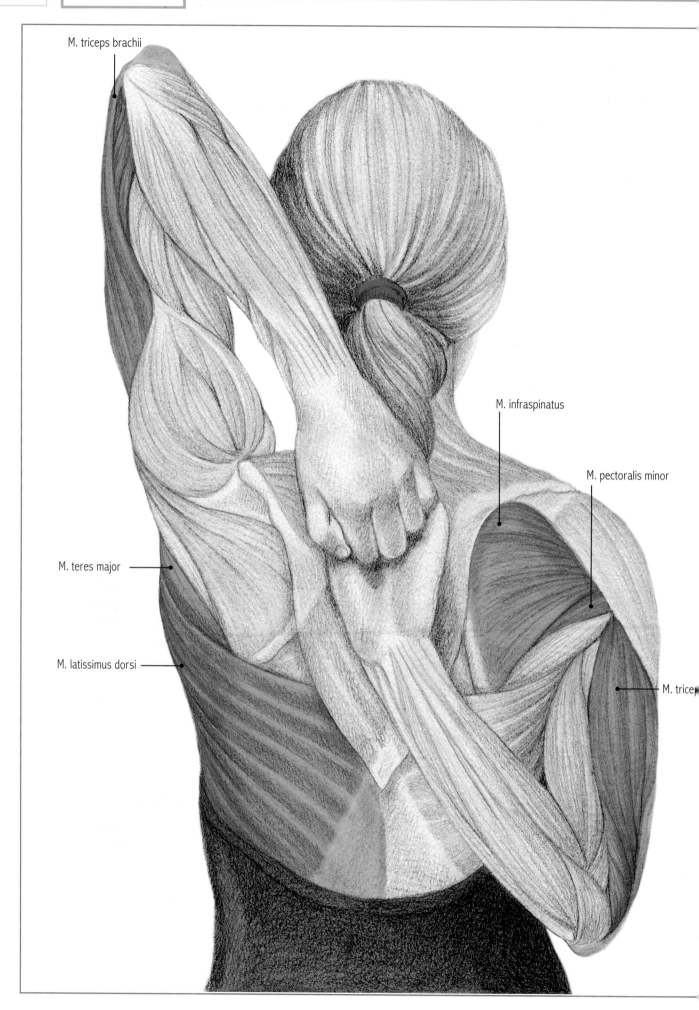

M. triceps brachii

M. infraspinatus

M. pectoralis minor

M. teres major

M. latissimus dorsi

M. trice

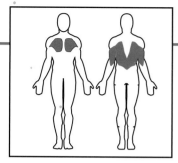

Muscles involved

Principal: External and internal rotators, triceps

Secondary: Pectoral, dorsal and teres major

Execution

This exercise is performed either standing, or seated in a back-less bench. Raise one arm over and behind the head while the other goes behind the back, and try to grab the fingers of both hands behind the upper back.

Comments

During this exercise, the mobility of the shoulder joint is quickly determined. Advanced trainers will have no difficulty linking their hands, and some may even grab the forearms. The rest should use some help in order to improve. This help could be in the form of a rope with knots that one can grab on to, and as time goes on and with increased practice, the person should be able to grab a knot that is progressively closer to the other hand. The help of a training partner can be very useful and it is very easy to do, standing behind the person doing the stretching and pushing gently upon the elbows in an effort to bring the hands closer together.

With each repetition, you should change the position of the arms in order to balance the stress upon the structures being stretched.

 It is true that the shoulders must not fall forward to form a hunched back, but neither should we obsessively force the posture and "throw our shoulders back" permanently. The body posture has to be relaxed. If one has a tendency to hunch over, it is frequently enough to simply elevate the chest slightly in order to adopt a better posture.

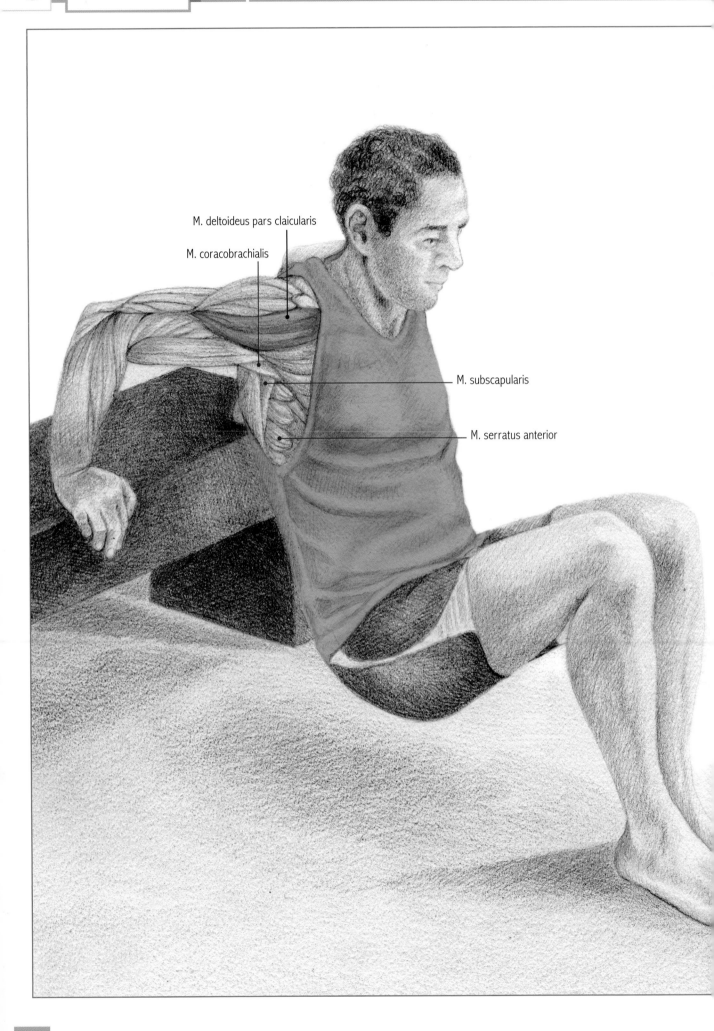

M. deltoideus pars claicularis

M. coracobrachialis

M. subscapularis

M. serratus anterior

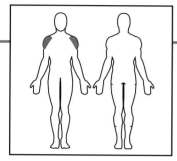

Muscles involved

Principal: Anterior deltoids

Secondary: Coracobrachialis, subscapularis, serratus

Execution

Sit horizontally on a flat bench with your hands on the edge of the bench. Separate yourself slightly from the bench in order to lower the torso down to the point where the arm forms a 90° angle. The soles of the feet must remain firmly in place, supporting the majority of the body weight.

Comments

This exercise stretches the muscles indicated, but having to support the body at the same time takes away from the effectiveness of the stretch itself. This can easily be understood if you think of the following. A muscle that is contracting cannot at the same time relax in order to be stretched. Therefore, the exercise may serve to distend the muscles indicated after a session of physical exercise, but not so much as a true stretching exercise during a session aimed at significantly improving mobility.

The name "dip on a bench" comes from the muscle-building exercise from which this stretch is derived, "dips on a bench." But this time, since it is not the movement but rather the position that is held, it is named in the singular. In contrast to the muscle building exercise, which targets the triceps and deltoids, here we want to place the emphasis predominantly on the anteriordeltoid.

Variation   3.2... With assistance holding on to a bar

To avoid the problem of the tension explained above, this variation is particularly effective. Sit on a flat bench, holding on to a wooden bar (or something similar) behind the back with a pronated grip (palms facing backward). A partner will pull upward on the bar, without separating it from your back, so that the elbows flex. The movement must be slow and controlled, otherwise it could injure the shoulder.

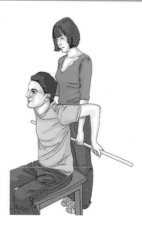

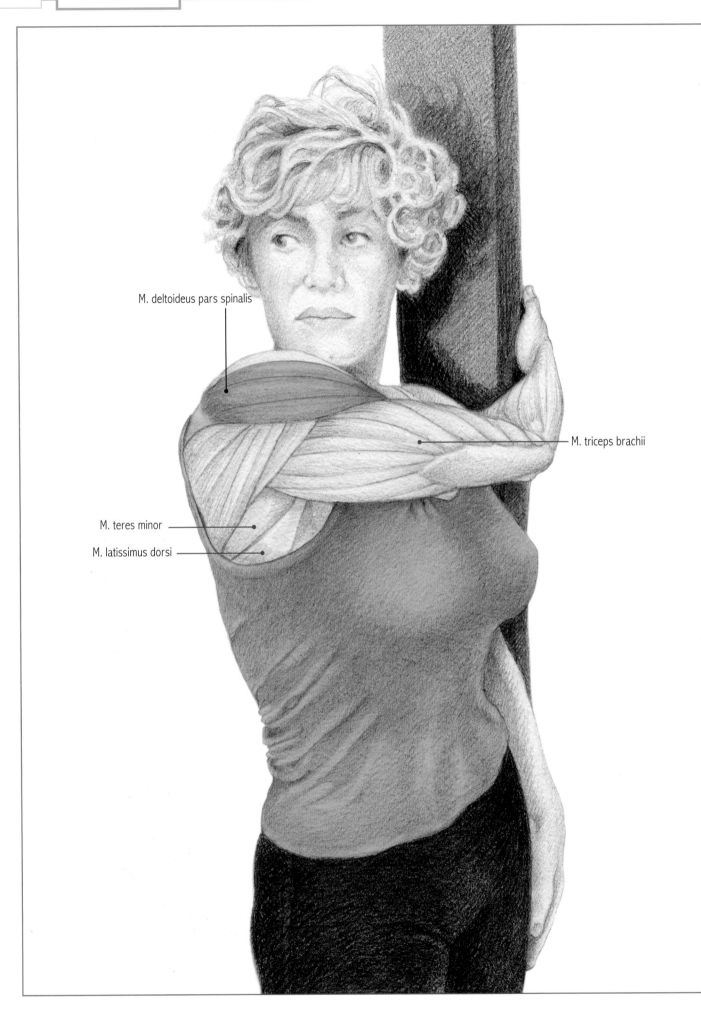

M. deltoideus pars spinalis

M. triceps brachii

M. teres minor

M. latissimus dorsi

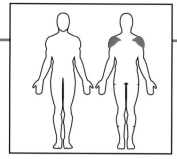

Muscles involved

Principal: Anterior deltoids

Secondary: Rhomboids, triceps, infraspinatus, teres minor, latissimus dorsi, teres major

Execution

Standing up next to a vertical bar, hold on to the bar with the arm located farther away from it. Turn the torso without letting go of the bar, so that you can feel the stretch along the back of the arm that is holding on to the bar.

Comments

This exercise is similar to the first one described in this chapter. This series of exercises is designed to stretch the rear portion of the shoulder and they are very beneficial for preventing the contractures that occassionaly develop in this area. And furthermore, they are a perfect complement to massages to eliminate contractures once they have developed. The only difficulty lies in not tensing the entire arm, but rather just the hand in its grip. The mental picture that we have to maintain to achieve this is thinking of the hands as just simple hooks that are fixed to immobilize them.

Keep the arm completely horizontal, with the hand gripping the bar at shoulder height, since this guarantees the optimum stretch of some of the muscles we are targetting, such as the rear deltoid and the rhomboids.

The exercise can also be done in pairs, who should stand far enough apart in order to be able to hold on to each other. However, it is much more effective when performed with a fixed support where one does not need to be concerned about exerting more or less tension than the other person.

Variation   **4.2... In quadruped position**

The same area that you are looking to stretch can be stretched from this position, in which, on your knees and supporting yourself with one arm, the other arm is passed underneath the body and pressure is exerted down upon it.

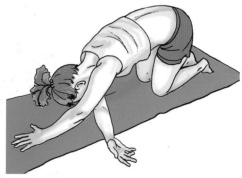

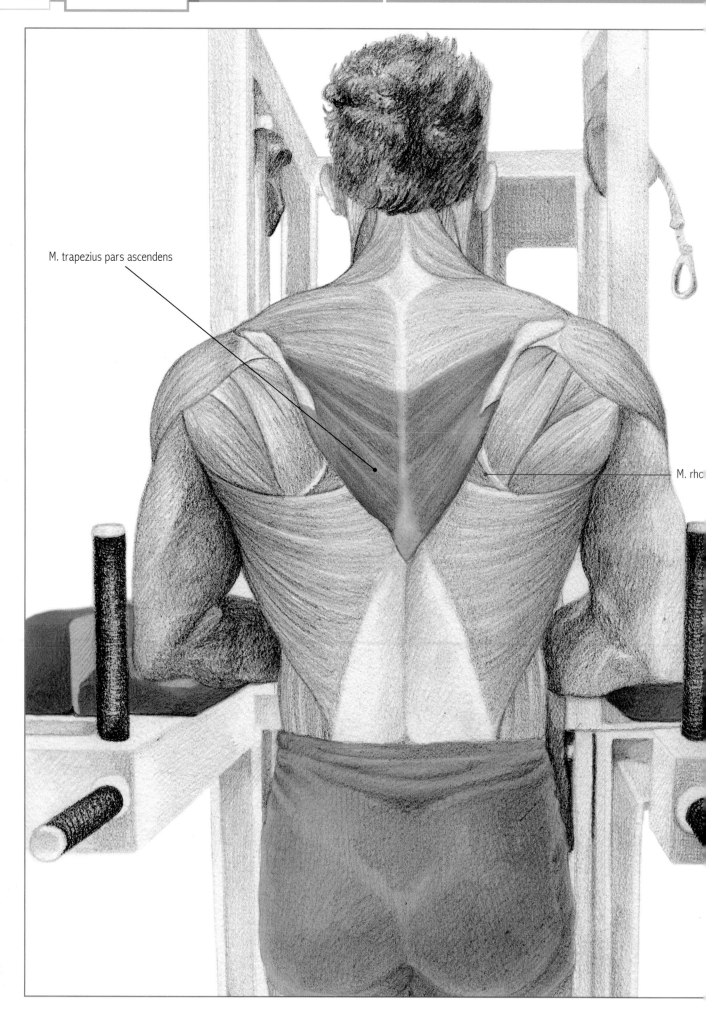

M. trapezius pars ascendens

M. rh[...]

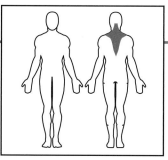

Muscles involved

Principal: Pectoralis minor, lower trapezius

Secondary: Rhomboids, serratus

Execution

Using a padded parallel apparatus, rest your elbows and forearms on the pads to support yourself and let your body hang down passively.

Comments

This is a very simple exercise that aims to stretch some muscles that are not regularly stretched by most conventional stretching exercises. However, the position is very limited for the joint mobility. In this posture, furthermore, the column is placed in a discharge position, which is very beneficial to alleviate any tensions that build up in it.

The head may be in line with the shoulders, but a greater stretch is achieved if the head is flexed slightly, allowing the shoulders to come up beside it.

Due to its simplicity, this exercise can be performed by both beginners and experienced individuals. People with columnar deviations, particularly scoliosis, should include this exercise in their repertoire.

 The simple fact of hanging in suspension from a bar implies a beneficial extension of the column, except for the cervical spine, which requires some sort of manual traction or another type of specific mobilization, since it is located above the arms.

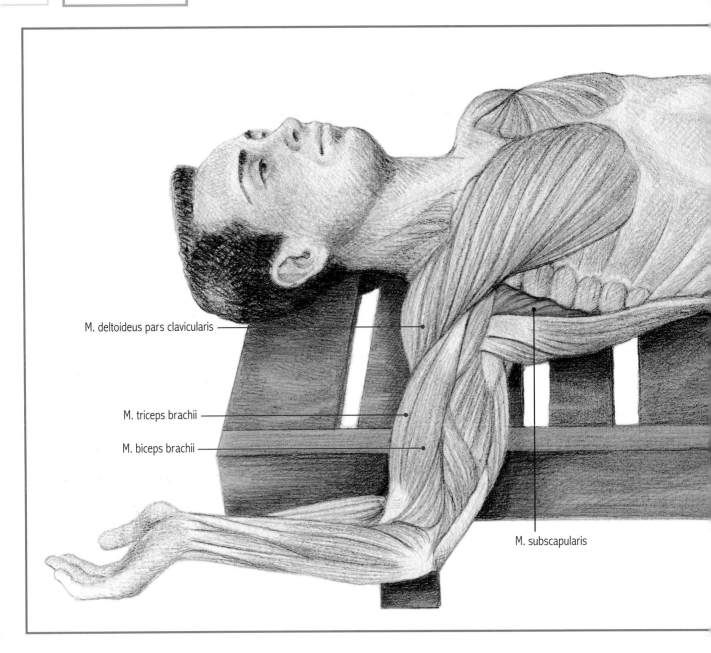

M. deltoideus pars clavicularis

M. triceps brachii

M. biceps brachii

M. subscapularis

Execution

Lying flat on your back (decubitus prone position) on a bench so that the arm that is going to be stretche overhangs from the side of the bench. Abduct the arm 90° and flex the elbow 90° as well. Now the arm should be perpendicular to the body, and the forearm should be perpendicular to the ground.. From tha position, externally rotate the arm. In other words, rotate the arm toward the back so that the palm of th hand is facing upward.

Comments

The set of rotator cuff muscles are vitally important for the stability of the shoulder joint, both in terms its strengthening as well as mobility. This exercise must be done gently, with the force of gravity providir enough tension to hold the position. In order to increase the tension, you can hold a small dumbbell in on hand (between 1 and 4 kg). In any case, you must be careful to slow the descent of the arm; only once yo have reached the final position can the muscles of the shoulder be relaxed so that it is gravity that is doir the stretching, but once again insisting on a controlled descent.

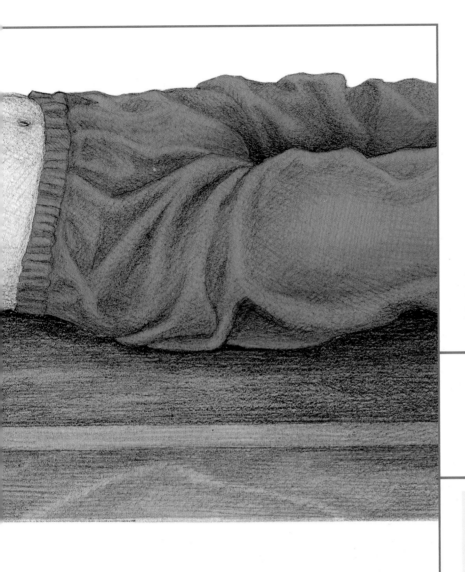

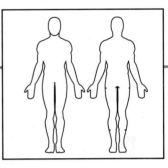

Muscles involved

Principal: Subscapularis

Secondary: Long head of the biceps, anterior deltoids

6.2... With internal rotation

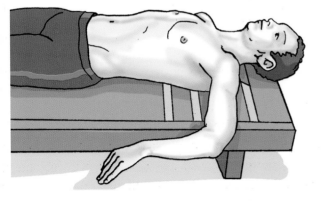

Principal: Infraspinatus

Secondary: Teres major, rear deltoids

Starting from an identical position, now the rotation is internal; in other words, the palm of the hand will end up facing the ground. The same precautions apply, and furthermore, with this particular variation, you need to pay particular attention that the shoulder does not come off the bench, which can easily occur unless we consciously prevent it.

It is advisable to alternate external and internal rotations of the arm, following the preceptive pause at the point of maximum stretch.

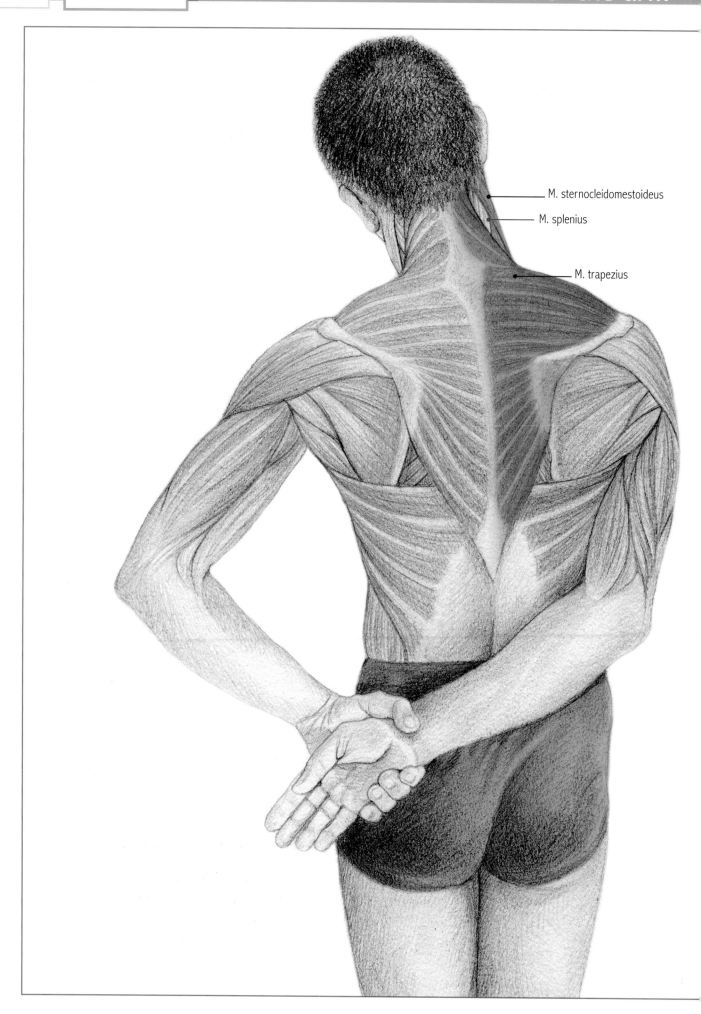

M. sternocleidomestoideus

M. splenius

M. trapezius

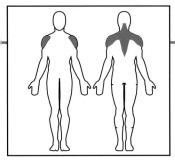

Muscles involved

Principal: Trapezius, sternocleidomastoid, levator scapulae, scalene

Secondary: Semispinalis, splenius, spinalis, splenius cervicis, occipitalis major and minor, multifidus, obliquus capitis major and minor, major and minor complexes, supraspinatus

Execution

Standing in front of a mirror, both arms are placed behind the back, one of them remains relaxed while the other pulls to its side. At the same time, allow the head to tilt slightly in the same direction that it is being pulled.

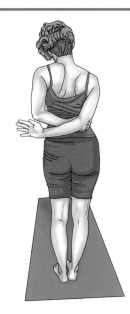

Comments

While performing this exercise, you should be able to feel the tension from the base of the skull to the arm. If you want to put more emphasis on the muscles of the shoulder, it is enough to simply not lean the head, or to tilt it to the side of the shoulder that is being stretched (that way the tension over certain muscles of the neck is nullified).

Similarly, it can be done by holding on to a vertical support with the arm that is being stretched. Alternatively, a partner could hold on to the arm while at the same time ensuring that, when the arm is pulled, the person being stretched does not flex the head to one side or lean the torso.

 Most people have a similar degree of joint mobility on both sides of their bodies. Professional athletes tend to be an exception. The specific characteristics of the sport in question can make one side of the body be more developed than the other. Logically, this does not occur with those sports where both sides of the body are equally exercised. This exception means that their training also needs to be very specific, requiring special strength and training exercises, and in some cases asymmetrical, in order to compensate. Some obvious examples are tennis, golf, shot putting, javelin throw, fencing, etc.

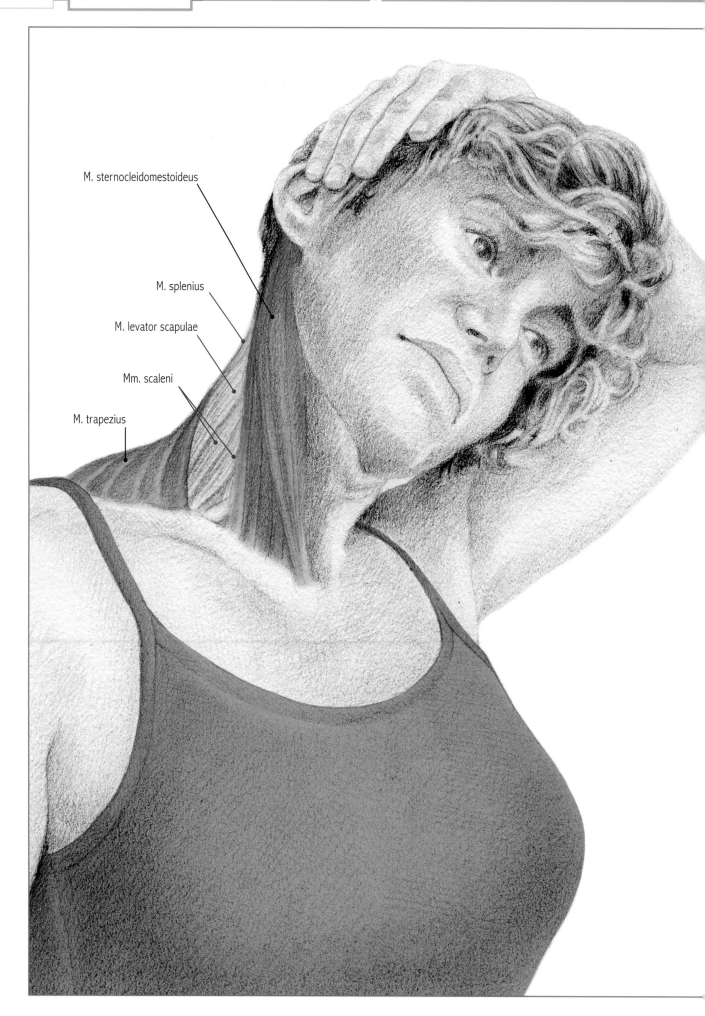

M. sternocleidomestoideus

M. splenius

M. levator scapulae

Mm. scaleni

M. trapezius

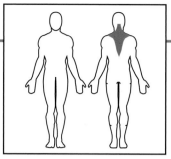

Muscles involved

Principal: Trapezius, sternocleidomastoid

Secondary: Scalene, semispinalis, splenius, spinalis, splenius cervicis, erectors, occipitalis major and minor, multifidus, obliquus capitis major and minor, levator scapulae, and major and minor complexes

Execution

Either standing or sitting down in front of a mirror, let your head tilt to one side, and then move it a few more degrees down with the help of the ipsilateral hand. As with all stretching exercises, and stretching exercises of the neck in particular, the movement must be slow and controlled.

Comments

With this exercise, you will quickly notice the tension on the side of the neck. If you wish to place less emphasis on this area and more on the posterior area, all you need to do is turn the head slightly, as if trying to look at the shoulder that is being stretched. Therefore, the range through which the head can be turned goes from looking straight ahead to looking at the shoulder.

If you elevate the shoulder on the side that is being stretched, you eliminate the stress upon certain muscles (e.g., the larger ones, such as the trapezius) while maintaining the tension on the small muscles of the cervical spine. On the other hand, there is the case of the arm pulling behind the back with the help of the other arm, so that the clavicular waist that is being stretched is always kept low, as is shown in exercise 7 of this chapter.

One last consideration is learning to perform the stretch of the cervical region all together. There is a tendency to tilt only the head, forgetting the more distal cervical vertebrae (the ones closer to the thoracic region).

 Although certain exercises may be performed standing up, seated or lying down, when it comes to the movements of the head, it is generally recommended that you do not do them standing up, so you avoid losing your balance. Furthermore, it should be kept in mind that it is not only the muscles and tendons that cross the joints in the neck (for example, the transverse processes of the first six cervical vertebrae are crossed by the vertebral artery, which supplies the brain.

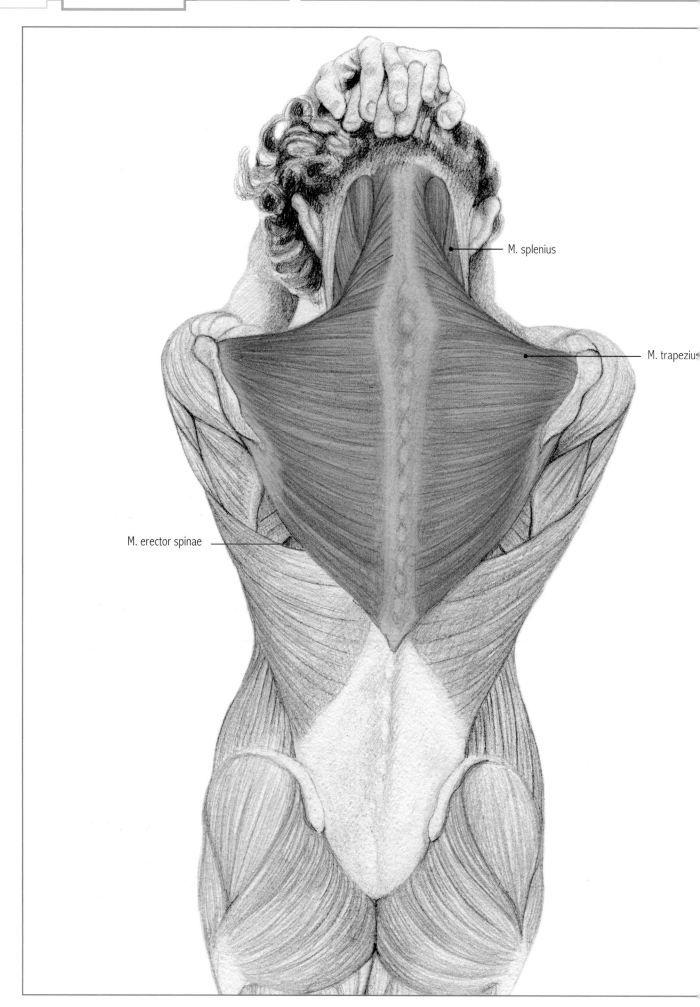

M. splenius

M. trapezius

M. erector spinae

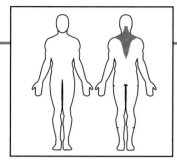

Muscles involved

Principal: Semispinalis, splenius, spinalis, splenius cervicis, spinal erectors, trapezius

Secondary: Occipitalis major and minor, multifidus, obliquus capitis major and minor, levator scapulae, major and minor complexes

Execution

Either standing or sitting down (preferably the latter) allow the head to fall gently forward in flexion, with the aid of both hands placed on top of each other in the occipital region of the head.

Comments

It is not necessary to apply force with the arms, since just their simple weight resting on the back of the head is enough. However, it may occur that the cervical muscles suddenly tense up to prevent the head from falling forward. To avoid that, the movement must be performed very slowly, and only at the very end of the movement should the entire area be relaxed to allow the force of gravity to be the one that performs the stretching. Meanwhile, the rest of the column must maintain its normal straightened posture.

To focus on the small extensor muscles of the head — and not so much on those of the vertebrae farther down — the turn must be done at the base of the skull with the chin close to the neck and gripping the head high with the hands.

The variation of this exercise where the neck is flexed in addition to the head is explained farther in this chapter (see exercise 12).

Variation   9.2... Lying down

The target position in this variation of the exercise is the same, except here we are lying down on a mat. The only difference is that now, it is not the force of gravity, but rather the force of the arms, that produces the stretching.

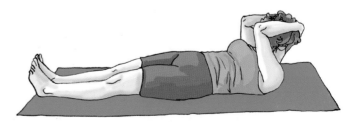

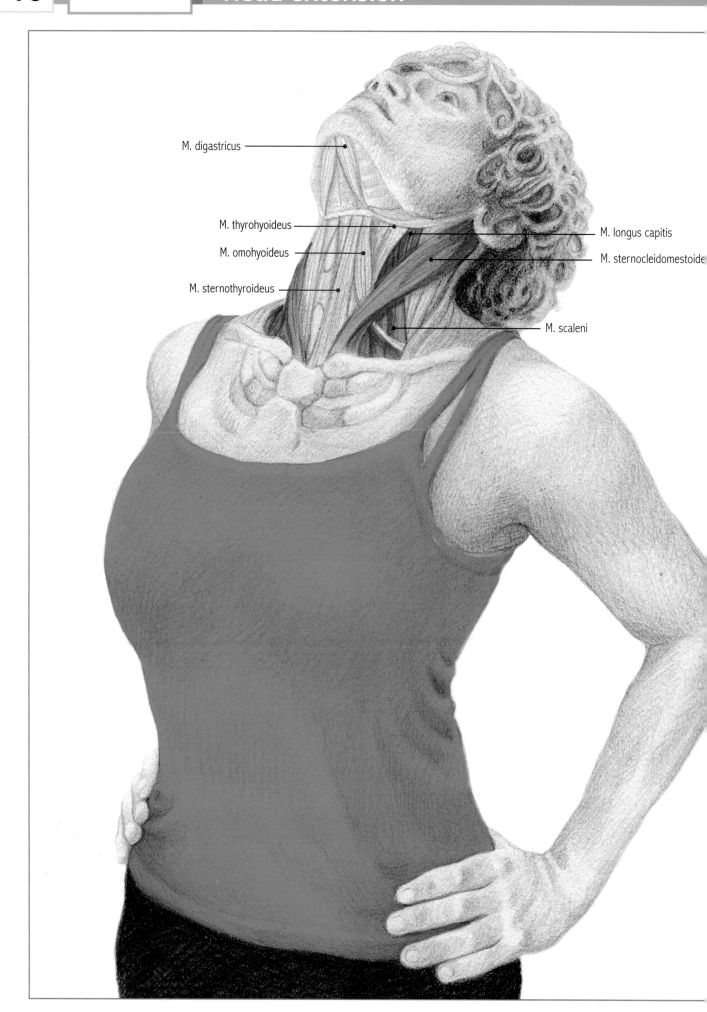

M. digastricus

M. thyrohyoideus

M. omohyoideus

M. sternothyroideus

M. longus capitis

M. sternocleidomestoide

M. scaleni

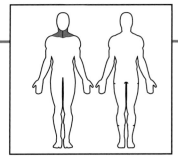

Muscles involved

Principal: Scalene, longissimus capitis and cervicis, anterior rectus, sternocleidomastoid

Secondary: Mylohyoid, thyrohyoid, sternocleidomastoid, sternohyoid, omohyoid

Execution

Either standing or sitting down (preferably the latter) on a high, back-less bench. Allow the head to fall gently backward in extension.

Comments

This exercise is much more delicate than the previous one where the head was flexed. What's more, if you suffer from any kind of cervical pain, it is better to not perform this exercise at all. In fact, some of the muscles that are stretched here are also stretched in movements that involve turning and leaning the head, both of which are much more comfortable movements than this one.

Placing the hands under the chin can help to complete the movement and achieve the posture that is indicated. As is the case with other exercises of the head, if you develop any headache or dizziness, this exercise can be eliminated from your repertoire or reduced to simple movements of mobility, without applying tension.

The jaw should remain closed if you want to involve a greater number of muscles in the exercise.

Variation   10.2... Lying down

For this exercise, lie down on a horizontal bench in such a way that the head hangs over the edge of the bench and simply allow gravity to extend the head. Although it may seem obvious, we will still point out that the movement needs to be performed in a very slow and controlled fashion.

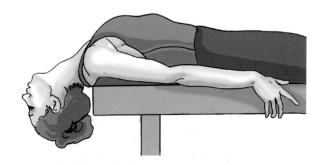

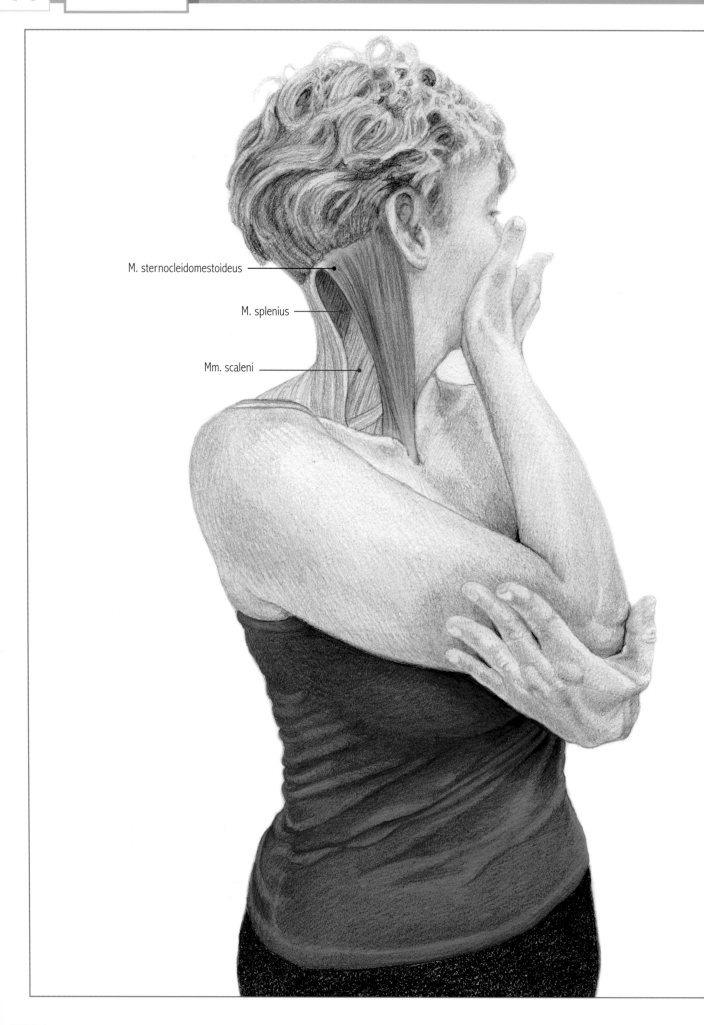

M. sternocleidomestoideus

M. splenius

Mm. scaleni

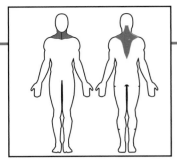

Muscles involved

Principal: Sternocleidomastoid, splenius

Secondary: Scalene, levator scapulae, posterior rectus major, obliquus capitis major and minor

Execution

Either standing or sitting down, turn the head to one side with the help of the opposite arm. The hand that helps with the turning will rest on the jaw, while the other hand will provide the push upon the elbow, as it is shown in the accompanying image.

Comments

The help of the arms is needed in order to be able to relax all of the cervical musculature and, in this way, perform the exercise correctly.

Although the tension in the superficial muscles of the area is evident, this exercise also serves to stretch the little muscles that surround the cervical spine and that, when they act unilaterally, assist in turning the head.

The variation of this exercise where the head is turned first to one side and then to the other, in an attempt to achieve a greater range of motion, is totally inadvisable. Any stretching for the neck muscles must be static, and in any case, never a "ballistic type" movement.

There are physiotherapy techniques in which a sharp turn of the head is performed in order to "align" certain cervical structures. Only qualified professionals should perform this movement.

 In addition to the slowness and the control with which exercises of the head and neck should be performed, and which we have repeatedly pointed out in several parts of the book, there is another consideration that must be kept in mind when stretching these areas: The stretching exercises must never be so prolonged or intense as in the rest of the body. In addition to being able to cause a headache and dizziness, they tend to be weaker structures and more sensitive than in other parts of the body.

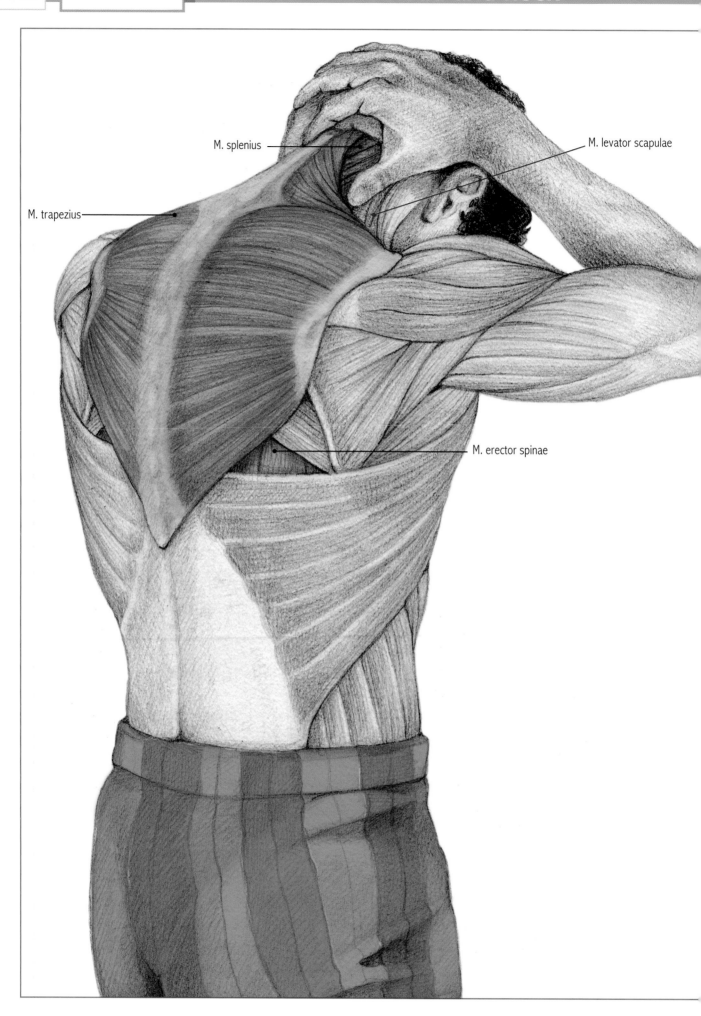

M. splenius

M. levator scapulae

M. trapezius

M. erector spinae

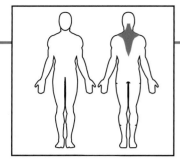

Muscles involved

Principal: Trapezius, semispinalis, splenius, spinalis, spinalis cervicis, spinal erectors

Secondary: Posterior rectus capitis major and minor, multifidus, obliquus capitits major and minor, levator scapulae, major and minor complexes

Execution

Seated or standing, take the head with the whole hand and flex downward and forward in a very gentle and sustained motion.

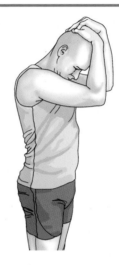

Comments

This exercise is very similar to one shown before (see exercise 9), but here it is not just a matter of flexing the head down (to stretch the small muscles of the back of the head) but rather to hold the head with the entire palm of the hand and thus pull it forward as well, in order to also stretch the larger muscles, such as the trapezius, as well as the lower areas of the cervical spine. As with all exercises of the head and neck, the movements should be especially slow and controlled.

This time, the tension will be felt in the lower cervical vertebrae, as well as in the muscles that surround the neck along the sides and back. The shoulders are not elevated, as this would reduce the effectiveness of the stretch.

If the flexion is accompanied by a turning of the head to one of the sides (bringing the cheek to the shoulder at the same time that the ipsilateral arm does the pulling), the focus will be on the extensor muscles of the opposite side, such as the splenius.

 After the mobilization exercises of the head and neck, and in the rests in between sets, it is recommended that you move the head in small lateral circles to facilitate relaxation.

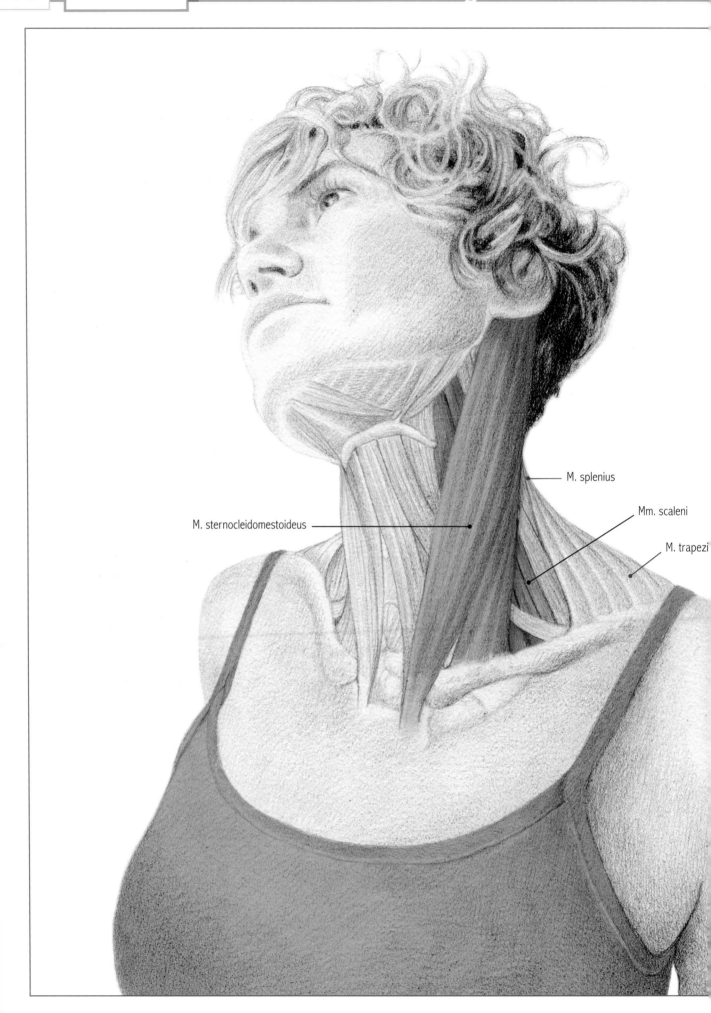

M. splenius

Mm. scaleni

M. trapezi

M. sternocleidomestoideus

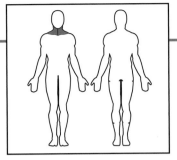

Muscles involved

Principal: Sternocleidomastoid, scalene, longissimus capitis, rectus anterior

Secondary: Hyoid group, splenius, semispinalis, spinalis, spinalis cervicis, erectors, multifidus, obliquus capitis major and minor, levator scapulae, major and minor complexes, trapezius

Execution

Standing up, or preferably sitting down, the head is leaned to one side and slightly rotated laterally. The movement is as if you were "looking at a top corner of the wall."

Comments

These two movements must be combined in order to be able to stretch a whole series of muscles within the complexity of the area being worked. Just as with other exercises of the head and neck, the movements should be slow and controlled, and the posture that you adopt must be a comfortable one.

If this exercise is performed correctly, then the tension in the muscles indicated is easily felt. One must avoid the error of leaning the body in order to locate the sights on the targeted area, since the movement should only be of the head and neck; the shoulders remain horizontal, relaxed. Should it be necessary, you may rest the hand from the opposite side upon the shoulder where the tension is being felt (over the clavicle), which will help to immobilize the shoulder and increase the stretching sensation.

 It is not only the muscles and tendons that are stretched during an exercise, the rest of the joint structures and even the skin, can be stretched as well. In fact, although it may not always be the case, at times it is these other structures that impose the limits on the stretching movements.

4

Biceps & Triceps Group

Descriptive anatomy of the flexor muscles of the arm: a biomechanical introduction to the principal muscles involved

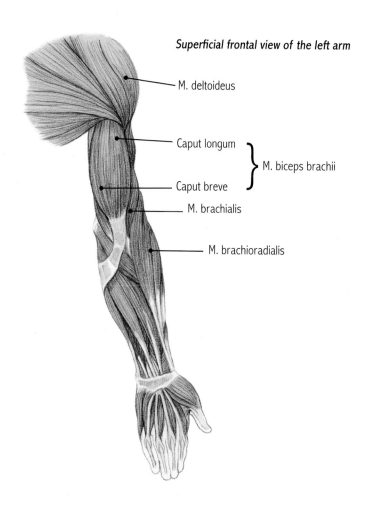

Superficial frontal view of the left arm

M. deltoideus

Caput longum
} M. biceps brachii
Caput breve

M. brachialis

M. brachioradialis

Biceps brachii (anterior, superficial)

Origin: Scapula (long head in the supraglenoid tubercle; short head in the coracoid process)

Insertion: Radius (radial tuberosity and bicipital-radial bursa)

Principal Functions: flexion of the elbow (especially in supination, both heads), and supination of the forearm (in flexion, both heads); abduction and medial rotation of the arm (long head); adduction (short head)

Brachioradialis/ long supinator (lateral, superficial)

Origin: Humerus (lateral suprachondylar border) and intermuscular plate

Insertion: Radius (external surface of the styloid process)

Principal functions: Flexion of the elbow (particularly in neutral and pronated positions) and returns the forearm to a neutral position from supination or pronation

Brachialis anterior (anterior, medial)

Origin: Humerus (distal half of its anterior face) and interosseo membrane

Insertion: Ulna (coronoid process tuberosity) and joint capsule

Principal functions: Pure flexion of the elbow (independently pronation/supination)

Brief comments: Almost everybody, including those who have never performed physical exercise in a systematic manner, knows an exercise that works the biceps. It is, without a doubt, the most popular muscle. But stretching it is somewhat different, in fact, since very few exercises are specific for the elbow flexors. Its anatomy, very limited in extension because of the bony encounters, is the reason why.

The brachioradialis is sometimes erroneously called "the long supinator," but a study of its anatomy reveals how inappropriate the pseudonym is.

Descriptive anatomy of the extensor muscles of the arm: a biomechanical introduction to the principal muscles involved

Triceps brachii (posterior, superficial)

Origin: Scapula (long head, in the infraglenoid tubercle), humerus (medial head, under the sulcus of the radial nerve; lateral head is proximal and lateral to the sulcus of the radial nerve, and extends proximally up to the point just below the greater tubercle)

Insertion: Ulna (olecranon) and posterior surface of the capsule

Principal functions: Extension of the elbow (all three heads), retroversion and adduction (long head)

Anconaeus (posterior, deep)

Origin: Humerus (dorsal surface of the lateral epicondyle) and external collateral ligament

Insertion: Ulna (proximal posterior one fourth, next to the triceps brachii).

Principal functions: Weak flexion of the elbow, tenses the joint capsule, minimal participation in supination/pronation

Brief comments: As is the case with the biceps and the brachialis, the extensors of the elbow also do not have a large variety of possible stretching exercises. Although in this case, the biarticular heads allow for a little more variety in the training, but a lot less than for other muscle groups, such as the legs, for example.

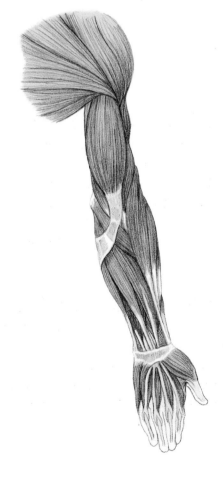

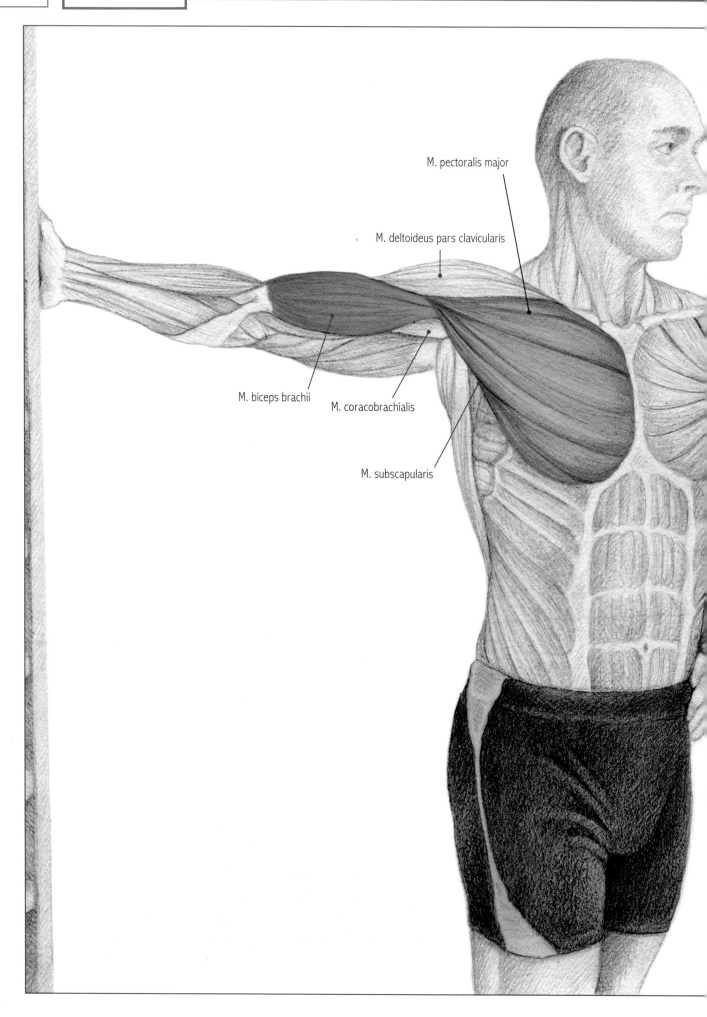

M. pectoralis major

M. deltoideus pars clavicularis

M. biceps brachii

M. coracobrachialis

M. subscapularis

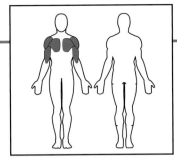

Muscles involved

Principal: Biceps, pectoralis major

Secondary: Anterior deltoids, coracobrachialis, subscapularis, pectoralis minor

Execution

Standing beside a wall or some other vertical support, raise the arm laterally (abduction), until shoulder height, with the palm of the hand turned so that it touches the frame of a door or the corner of a wall. The elbow remains extended. The arm and the pectoral region are relaxed, and the torso is then rotated in the opposite direction of the arm that is raised.

Comments

This exercise is performed in a similar way to that for the pectoral region, which was detailed in the corresponding chapter, but now the elbow must remain extended in order to achieve a good stretch of the biceps.

The person executing this movement must know how to feel the tension in the muscle that is being stretched, in this case the biceps brachii; otherwise, he may feel this tension somewhere else, perhaps in the pectoral region) and think that he or she is performing the exercise correctly. In this case, the person should modify the posture and begin the stretch again until he achieves the desired objective.

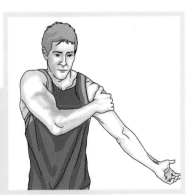

 The stretching of certain muscles involves an added degree of difficulty; the meeting of bony structures. The biceps is a clear example; once the elbow is extended, we have to rotate the forearm and move the shoulder in order to separate the muscle`s points of insertion.

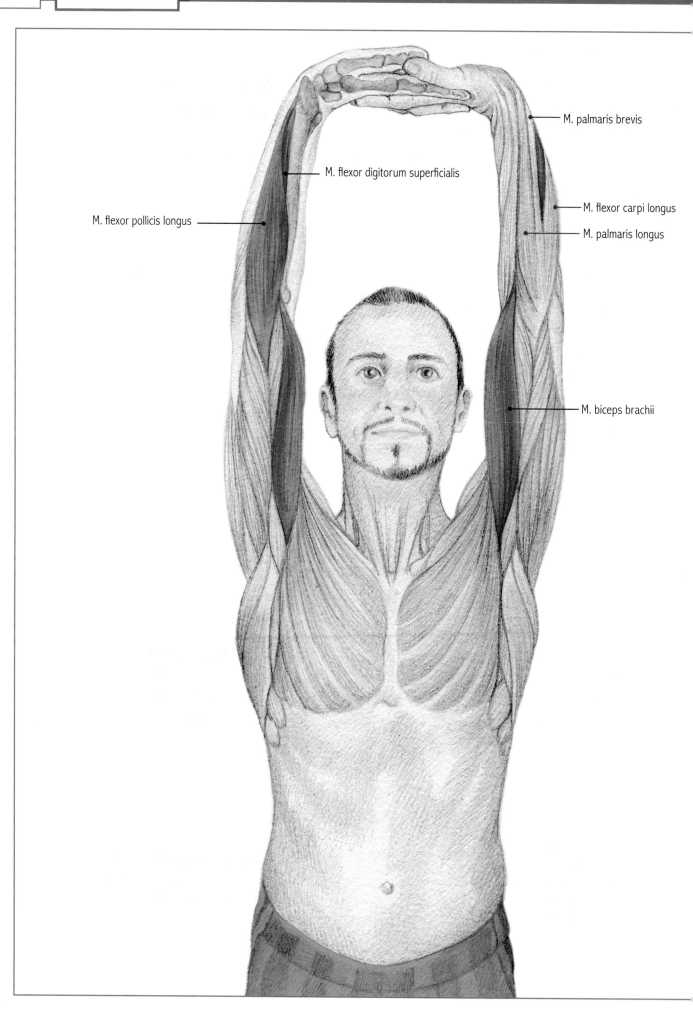

M. palmaris brevis

M. flexor digitorum superficialis

M. flexor pollicis longus

M. flexor carpi longus

M. palmaris longus

M. biceps brachii

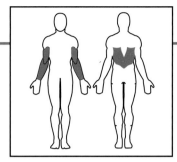

Muscles involved

Principal: Biceps brachii, flexor digitorum profundus and superficialis, flexor hallucis longus

Secondary: Anterior ulna, palmaris major and minor, latissimus dorsi, teres major

Execution

Standing up or sitting in front of a mirror, elevate the arms above the head in complete extension. The palm of one hand is placed under the back of the other hand because if the fingers were interlaced, then the extension of the elbow would be limited at the point of maximum stretch for the finger and wrist flexors.

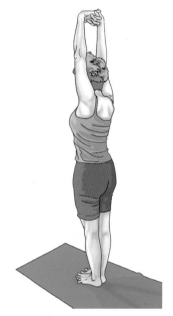

Comments

As with other stretching exercises for the biceps, the one that is detailed here does not achieve a maximum stretch of said muscle, and thus should not be the only exercise performed for the purpose of stretching the biceps. It is necessary to add more variety if what we want is to truly stretch this muscle.

We can classify this exercise as one of mobility and for getting the stiffness out, more than as an exercise to improve the flexibility of the biceps.

 Everyone knows that the biceps flexes the arm, since it is probably the best-known muscle. But in addition to this important function it is also a supinator of the forearm and it assists in the flexion of the shoulder, and as well as shoulder abduction and adduction, depending on whether its long head or its short head is more involved. It is even involved in the internal rotation of the arm.

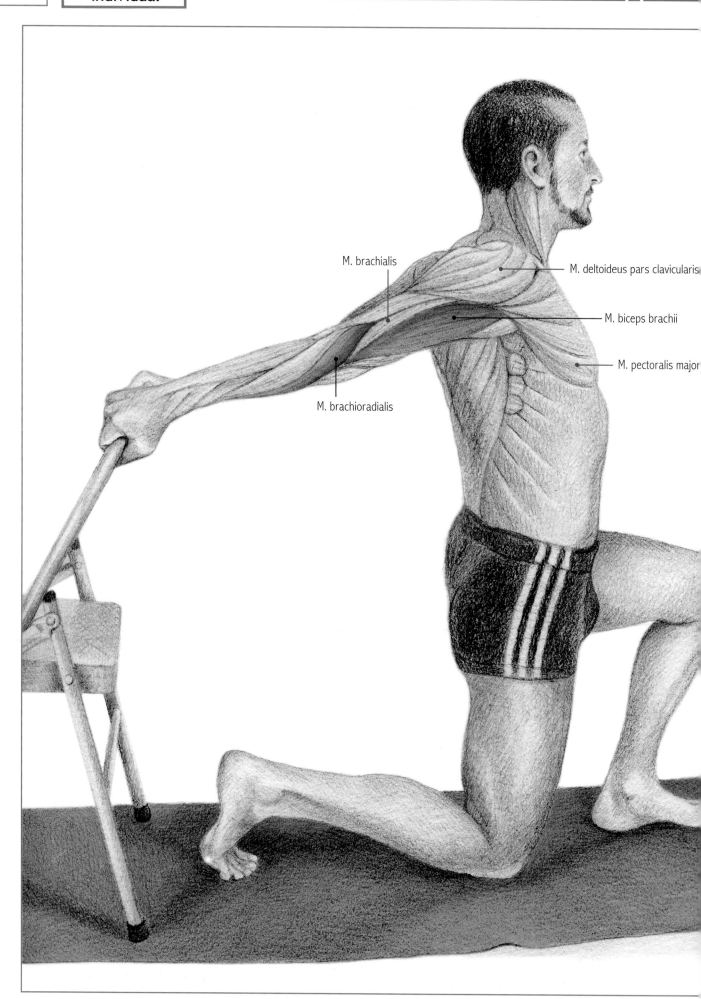

M. brachialis

M. deltoideus pars clavicularis

M. biceps brachii

M. pectoralis major

M. brachioradialis

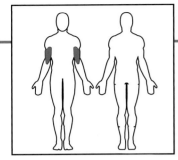

Muscles involved

Principal: Biceps brachii, brachioradialis

Secondary: Anterior brachial, pectoralis major, anterior deltoids, subscapularis

Execution

Standing up, with your back toward a fixed support of approximately shoulder-height, with the elbow extended and the arm internally rotated (with the thumb pointing inward), rest the back of the hand on the support and lower the trunk until you can feel the stretch in the area of the biceps.

Comments

As with other exercises, it is not enough to simply extend the elbow in order to stretch the biceps, you also have to move the shoulder to separate its points of insertion. This exercise manages a good stretch of the biceps, although like many others, it should be performed slowly. In fact, from among the exercises designed to stretch the biceps individually (without the help of a partner) this is one of the most effective.

Due to the position of the arm and the movement that we perform, the shoulder – particularly the anterior portion – is also stretched.

* In very muscular individuals, the complete flexion of the elbow is not possible, since the muscle masses from the arm and the forearm come together before full flexion is achieved. A partial solution is to try to relax the muscles that meet and exert pressure with the opposite arm, although to achieve this, it is preferable to perform this exercise with the help of a training partner (i.e., passive stretching).

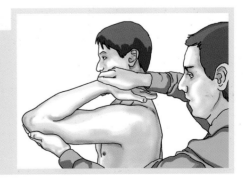

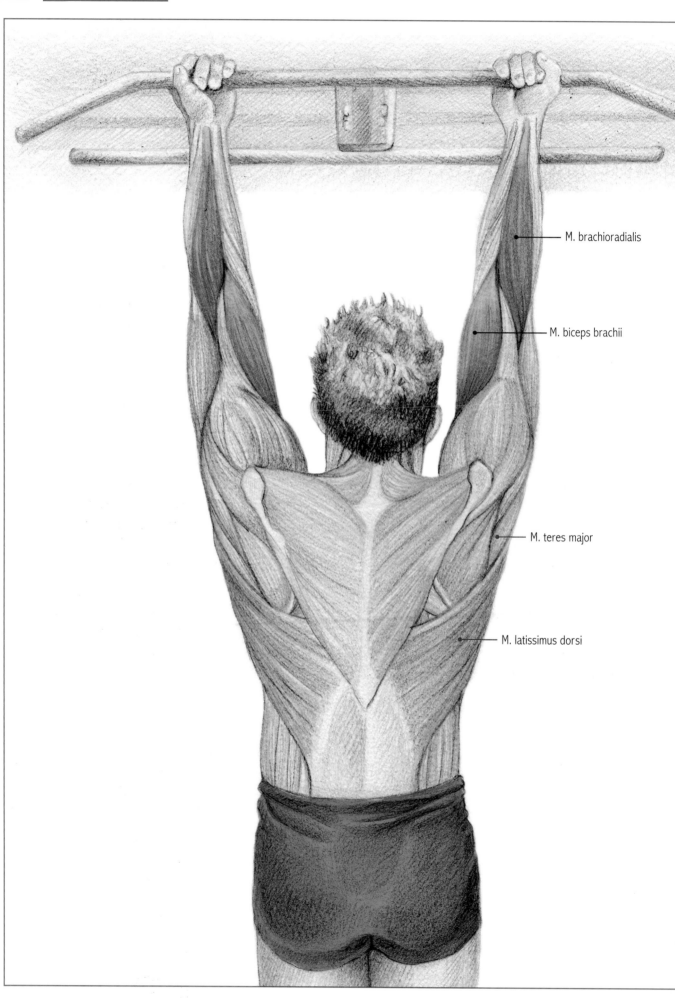

M. brachioradialis

M. biceps brachii

M. teres major

M. latissimus dorsi

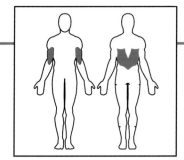

Muscles involved

Principal: Biceps brachii, brachioradialis

Secondary: Latissimus dorsi, teres major

Execution

With the arms externally rotated and the forearms supinated (with the palm of the hand facing backward), hang suspended from a horizontal bar. Relax the body during the few seconds that the stretch lasts and then we return to the ground in order to "release" the muscles.

Comments

This exercise is the starting position for performing "chin-ups" for the back and biceps. It is precisely this pair of muscle groups, the back muscles and the elbow flexors, that are stretched during this exercise. It is a very simple stretching exercise, which can be performed by just about anyone. The only particular points are knowing how to relax the body and not to maintain a constant tension in the arms, which would prevent them from being stretched, and use only the forearms and hands to support the weight of the body.

If there is not a bar available that is sufficiently high so as to allow the entire body to hang free, or if the person does not feel capable of doing so, he may hold on to a lower bar and keep the feet on the ground, but he must know how to progressively take all of the body weight off his feet until his whole bodyweight is hanging although his feet may still be touching the ground. If he is unable to do this, he must opt for the variation that is explained below.

Variation	4.2... On a pull-down machine

Those people who have a difficult time supporting their own body from a bar may find the solution in this exercise, because when using a machine, we can select the weight with which we want the machine to "pull" us in "passive traction."

Although we may find different types of grips with this type of machine, the best grip for stretching the biceps is on the straight bar with the writsts supinated (with the thumbs out to the sides).

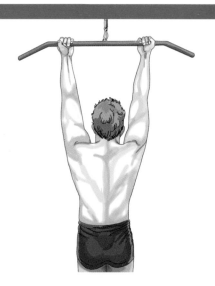

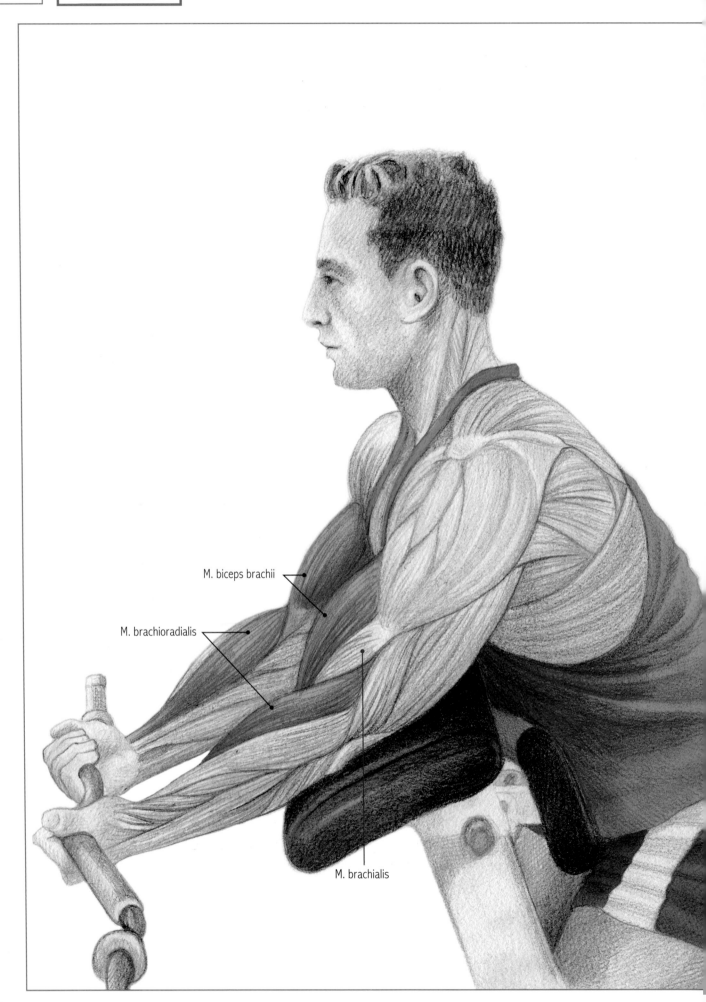

M. biceps brachii

M. brachioradialis

M. brachialis

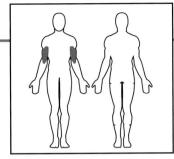

Muscles involved

Principal: Biceps brachii, brachioradialis

Secondary: Brachialis anterior

Execution

Sitting on the preacher bench, hold a bar with a supinated grip (palms facing upward), lean your elbows against the pads and let the arms extend until they reach the point of maximum extension.

To finish, it is not recommended that you simply return the weight up by flexing the elbows, but rather that you get up from the bench completely, so that it is more comfortable and less compromising for the joint.

Comments

Two comments need to be made concerning this exercise. On the one hand, although we are using an apparatus that is a classic in weightlifting gyms, this is a stretching exercise and you should not load the bar with too much weight. The extension should be slow and controlled, because otherwise the joint could be damaged at the bottom of the movement; maybe not the biceps itself, but the olecranon, the joint capsule, the humeral artery or certain ligaments.

For those people who find that the regular bar (which weights approximately 8 to 10 kg) is too much weight, they may look for a lighter bar, but never use dumbbells because it would be much harder to maintain full supination of the forearms, which is necessary for stretching the biceps.

One last reminder: the biceps is not the most pure flexor of the arm; the brachialis anterior is.

 Do stretches inhibit progress in the training for muscle hypertrophy? No. In fact, the greatest bodybuilding champions tend to have good flexibility, although their mobility may be somewhat limited by their bulk. It all depends on the type and the variety of training that is performed.

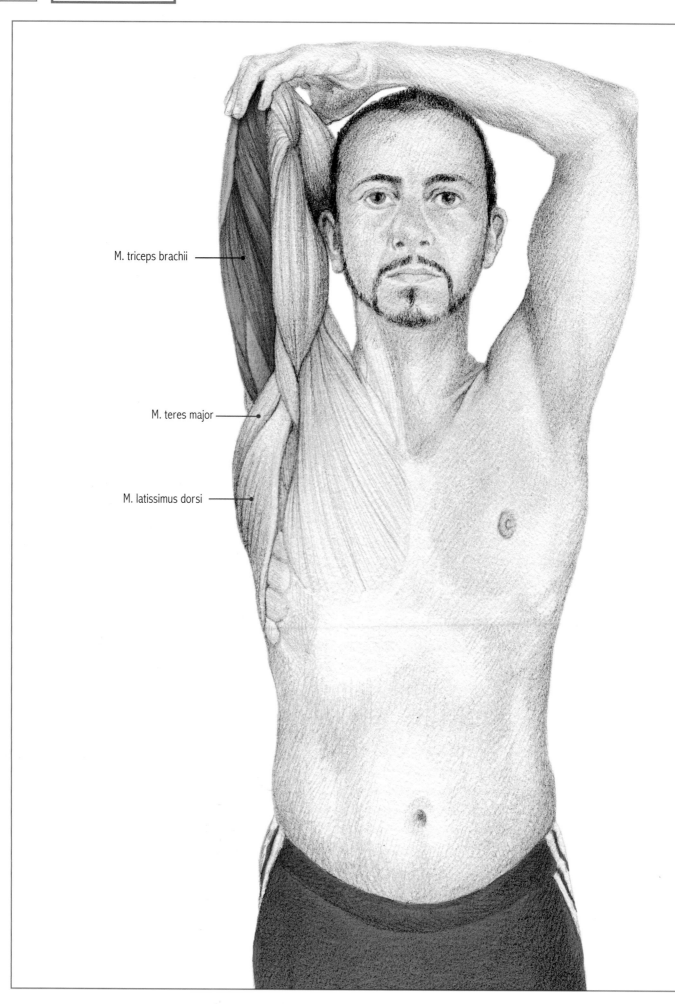

M. triceps brachii

M. teres major

M. latissimus dorsi

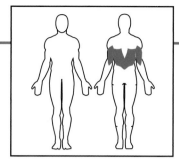

Muscles involved

Principal: Triceps brachii

Secondary: Latissimus dorsi, teres major, anconeus

Execution

Either standing up or sitting down in front of a mirror, flex the elbow maximally and raise the arm by flexing the shoulder while the opposite hand is used to push the elbow backward.

Comments

There is a tendency to rest the helping arm on the head as a kind of lever, which could force the cervical vertebrae. While this help could be useful if it is done correctly (since one has to withstand significant tension with the arm that is pushing on the elbow), care must be taken not to adopt poor postures with the neck.

It is imperative that the elbow is flexed maximally (hence the reason for naming this exercise hyperflexion, even if it is not literally accurate), yet it is not uncommon to see people who, as they push farther back, the elbow joint is progressively relaxed and extended, taking away from the stretching of the triceps.

Although the little soleus is also stretched in this exercise, this muscle does not need the movements of the shoulder to exercise it, and it would be enough simply with the deep flexion of the elbow, without modifying the position of the shoulder.

The help of a training partner is simple — all he has to do is ensure that the elbow remains totally flexed and push gently on it toward the back. It is more comfortable when the partner sits on a bench to receive the help. There are also those who prefer the bench (with a back support) when stretching alone since it is easier to keep one`s balance and focus on the exercise.

Variation   6.2... Over a support

The position now requires you to stand, but facing a bar or some other vertical support, which will serve as a support on which to push your body. Try to keep the elbow always maximally flexed. With respect to everything else, there are no diff erences between the exercises, except that it is much easier to push with the whole body, as is the case here, than with just the opposite hand (as is the case with the main exercise here), which could turn out to be much more comfortable for many trainees.

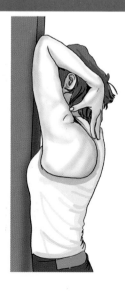

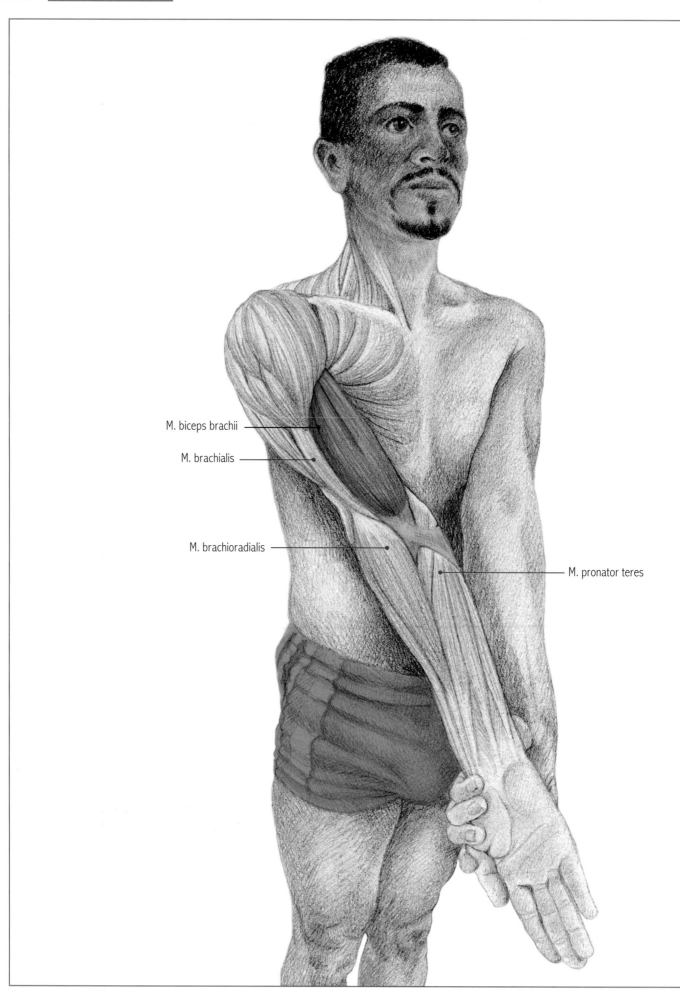

M. biceps brachii

M. brachialis

M. brachioradialis

M. pronator teres

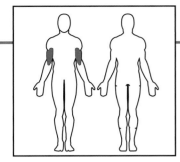

Muscles involved

Principal: Biceps brachii

Secondary: Coracobrachialis, branchialis anterior, pronators, brachioradialis

Execution

Stand before a mirror, stretch the elbow and force the pronation of the forearm with your other hand.

Comments

The pronation of the forearm helps to further separate the points of insertion of the heads of the biceps, although as it occurs with other stretching exercises for this muscle, the effects that are achieved are not very remarkable.

Although we have repeatedly pointed out in this chapter the impossibility inherent in finding optimal exercises for stretching the biceps, what is true is that this muscle does not require more demanding stretches, as it works well within the regular ranges of motion, and rarely encounters abnormalities in its mobility (which are much more frequent with many other muscles).

 One must not confuse pronation with the internal rotation of the shoulder, nor supination with external rotation. To better understand the movements of pronation / supination, it is better to perform them with the elbow flexed (consult the dictionary at the end of the book).

5

Forearms & Hands Group

Descriptive anatomy of the forearm: biomechanical introduction to the principal muscles

Superficial back view

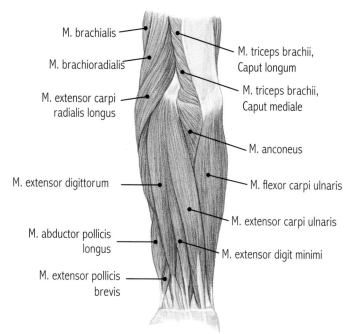

M. brachialis

M. brachioradialis

M. extensor carpi radialis longus

M. extensor digittorum

M. abductor pollicis longus

M. extensor pollicis brevis

M. triceps brachii, Caput longum

M. triceps brachii, Caput mediale

M. anconeus

M. flexor carpi ulnaris

M. extensor carpi ulnaris

M. extensor digit minimi

Superficial frontal view

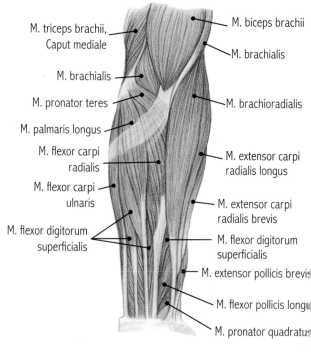

M. triceps brachii, Caput mediale

M. brachialis

M. pronator teres

M. palmaris longus

M. flexor carpi radialis

M. flexor carpi ulnaris

M. flexor digitorum superficialis

M. biceps brachii

M. brachialis

M. brachioradialis

M. extensor carpi radialis longus

M. extensor carpi radialis brevis

M. flexor digitorum superficialis

M. extensor pollicis brevis

M. flexor pollicis longu

M. pronator quadratus

Flexors

Flexor digitorum superficialis (anterior, superficial)

Origin: Humerus (epitrochlea) and radius (anterior medial surface), frequently also the cubitus (coronoid processes)

Insertion: Middle phalanges of the 2nd to 5th fingers

Principal functions: Strong flexion of the fingers and wrist, weak elbow flexion

Flexor carpi ulnaris / anterior ulnar (anterior-medial, superficial)

Origin: Humerus (epitrochlea) and cubitus (olecranon and the upper ulnar two-thirds; forearm fascia

Insertion: Pisiform, hook and 5th metacarpal

Principal functions: Palmar flexion and ulnar adduction. Collaborates in the flexion of the elbow

Pronator teres (anterior, superficial)

Origin: Humerus (medial epicondyle), cubitus (coronoid processes) and medial intermuscular septum

Insertion: Radius (medial and lateral portions of the radius)

Principal functions: Pronation of the forearm, flexion of the elbow

Flexor digitorum profundus (anterior, deep)

Origin: Cubitus (two-thirds of its palmar surface) and interosse membrana

Insertion: 2nd to 5th fingers (base of the terminal phalanges)

Principal functions: Flexion of the wrist and the carpal, metacar and phalangeal joints

Flexor carpi radialis / Palmaris major (anterior, superficial)

Origin: Humerus (epitrochlea) and superficial antebrachial fascia

Insertion: 2nd metacarpal (palmar surface of its base) a sometimes the 3rd

Principal functions: Weak flexion and pronation, also participates the flexion and radial abduction of the hand

Pronator quadratus (anterior, deep)

Origin: Cubitus (distal one-fourth of the anterior surface)

Insertion: Radius (distal one-fourth of the anterior surface)

Principal functions: Pronation

Imaris longus / minor (antero-medial, superficial)

Origin: Humerus (epitrochlea) and sometimes the forearm

Insertion: Palmar aponeurosis of the hand

Principal functions: Flexion of the hand and tenses the palmar aponeurosis, collaborates in the flexion of the elbow

Flexor pollicis longus (anterior, deep)

Origin: Radius (anterior surface)

Insertion: Thumb (base of the terminal phalanx)

Principal functions: Flexion and adduction of the last phalanx of the thumb

Brief comments: We generally have two uses for the hands (and forearms), strong gripping and fine manipulation. In both cases, we highly employ a whole series of muscles from those areas that, with overuse, can cause pain. Stretching the hands and the forearms is simple, they don`t require complicated postures and it can be done in any regular place. Taking a brief rest from the daily activities to dedicate a few minutes to the stretching of these areas can serve to prevent problems derived from their intense use.

Extensors

Extensor digitorum (posterior-medial, superficial)

Origin: Humerus (lateral epicondyle), external collateral ligament, anular ligament of the radius and antebrachial fascia

Insertion: 2nd to 5th fingers, with extensions up to the base of the proximal phalanges and the metacarpophalangeal joint capsules

Principal functions: Extension and adduction of the fingers, powerful extension of the wrist

Extensor carpi radialis brevis (posterior-radial, superficial)

Origin: Humerus (common head of the muscles of the lateral epicondyle of the humerus), external collateral ligament and anular ligament of the radius

Insertion: 3rd metacarpal (on its posterior base)

Principal functions: Dorsal flexion of the hand and takes the hand to medial position from ulnar adduction, weak elbow flexor

Extensor carpi radialis longus (lateral, superficial)

Origin: Humerus (lateral supracondylar border), intermuscular plate, lateral epicondyle

Insertion: 2nd metacarpal (on its posterior base)

Principal functions: Supination if extended, extension and radial abduction of the hand, weak elbow flexion

Extensor carpi ulnaris (posterior, superficial).

Origin: Humerus (epicondyle) and cubitus (medial third of the posterior border)

Insertion: 5th metacarpal (on its posterior base)

Principal functions: Ulnar adduction, extension of the wrist

Brachioradialis (lateral, superficial)

See "BICEPS"

Adductor policis longus

Cubitus to radius, crest of the supinator and interosseous membrane. Abduction of the thumb, palmar flexion and radial abduction.

Opponens policis

Trapezius and transverse carpal ligament to first metacarpal. Opposition of the thumb.

Extensor policis brevis

Cubitus and radius to thumb. Extension and abduction of the thum

Brief comments: All of the comments that were made on the "flexors" also apply to the extensors. In particular, we will note the strong use that is made of these little muscles in activities that, up to a few years ago, did not exist, such as those that are required to use a computer. It is precisely in these activities that the regular practice of stretching exercises best demonstrates its benefits.

On the other hand, a brief anatomical reminder is in order: there are no muscles per se in the wrists, but rather the muscles that pass through its tendons. Therefore, it is the insertion points in the forearm and in the fingers that are the determining factors in stretching exercises. This means that, when a stretching exercise is performed, it is not enough to simply focus on the position of the wrist, but also on the position of the elbow and fingers. There is an enormous difference, for example, between flexing the wrist when making a fist and flexing it when the hand is open.

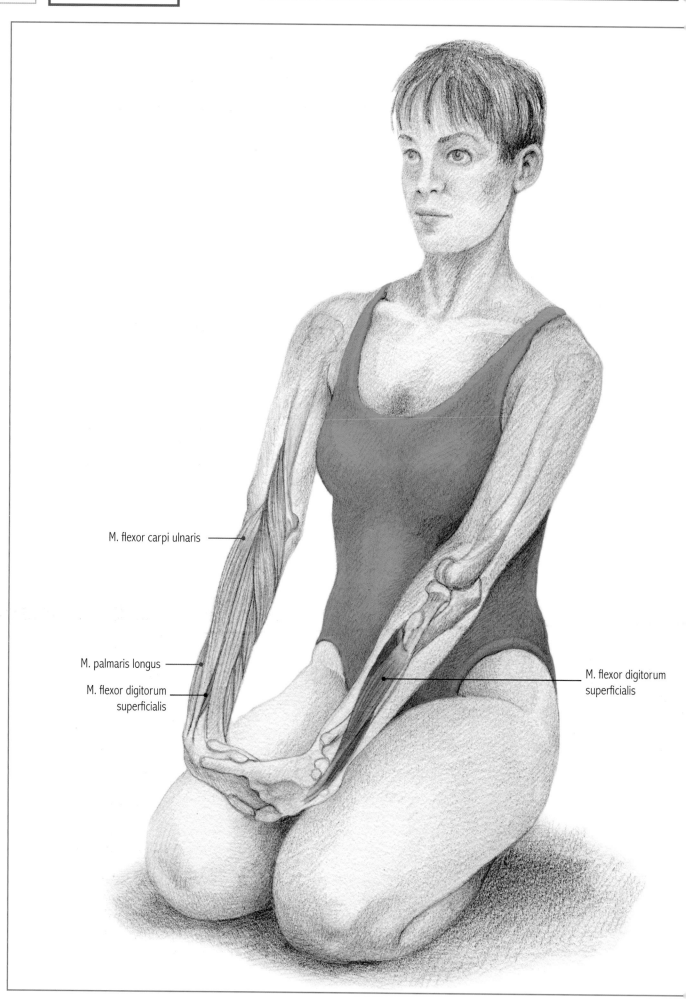

M. flexor carpi ulnaris

M. palmaris longus

M. flexor digitorum superficialis

M. flexor digitorum superficialis

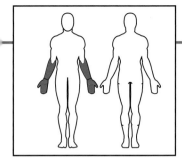

Muscles involved

Principal: Flexors of the fingers (deep, superficial, and the long flexor of the thumb)

Secondary: Anterior ulnar, palmaris major and minor

Execution

Interlace the fingers, with the palms facing each other, turn the forearms and extend the elbows toward the front. As you approach maximum extension of the elbows, you will feel the tension in the anterior part of the forearms.

Comments

This is a very simple exercise, very appropriate for any person who works intensely with the hands: information technology, construction worker, etc.

Variations

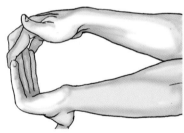

1.2 ... One hand helps the other

The position is similar, but now it is one hand that pulls the fingers of the other hand to provoke the extension of the wrist. There is significant tension placed on the flexor of the fingers and to do it in a uniform fashion, it is important to pull equally on all the fingers at the same time. A light extension of the wrist increases the tension.

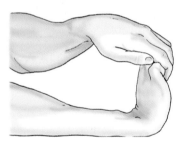

1.3 ... With the hand closed

Once again, the opposite hand to the one being stretched pulls on the fingers, but this time, the other hand remains semi-open, emphasizing the lumbrical muscles.

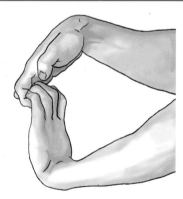

1.4 ... With the hand semi-open and pulling on the fingers

Identical position as in the previous variation, with the one exception that now the fist remains closed, achieving more emphasis on the anterior ulnar and the palmar muscles.

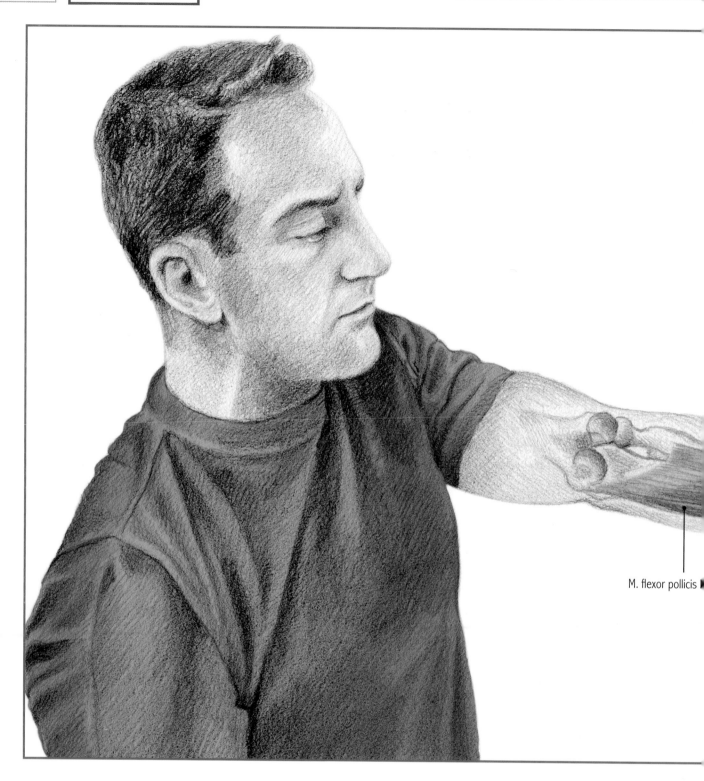

M. flexor pollicis ▶

Variations   **2.2 ... In quadruped**

On all fours on a lightly padded surface, place the arms in the way that is indicated in the main exercise, and lean the torso slightly backwards until you feel the tension in the forearms. The movement should be slow and gentle to avoid any injuries.

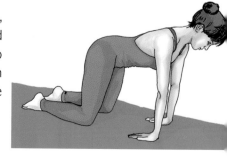

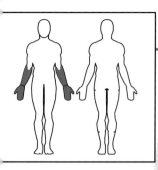

Muscles involved

Principal: Flexors of the fingers (deep, superficial, and the long flexor of the thumb)

Secondary: Anterior ulnar, palmaris major and minor

Execution

Stand in front of a wall with the arms extended and the tip of the fingers pointing downward, press lightly to the front until the entire palm of the hand is resting on the wall. The arms should be raised until almost shoulder height.

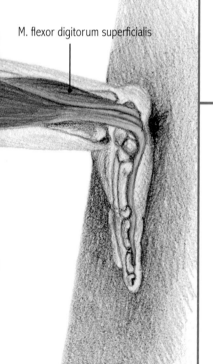

M. flexor digitorum superficialis

Comments

If the elbows are extended, it will stretch all of the muscles of the anterior part of the forearm, whereas if they remain partly flexed, the effort is centered on the small flexor muscles of the hand and fingers.

The way to increase the intensity is to place the hands somewhat higher on the wall and then press lightly as was previously explained.

2.3... Seated

To be more comfortable, sit and place the hands behind the body, and then move the trunk backwards until you can feel the tension in the forearms.

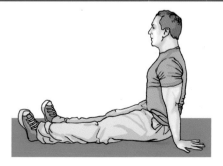

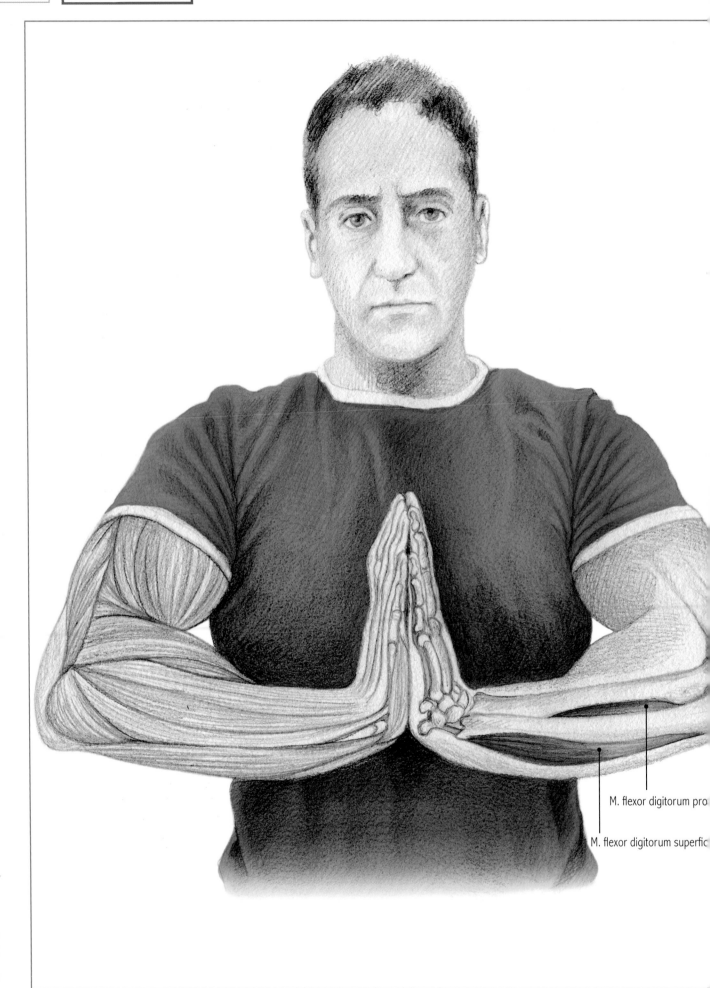

M. flexor digitorum pro

M. flexor digitorum superfic

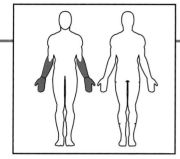

Muscles involved

Principal: Flexor digitorum profundus, abductor pollicis, flexor policis longus

Secondary: Flexor digitorum superficialis, anterior ulnar, palmaris major and minor

Execution

Stand or sit, preferably in front of a mirror, place the hands with the palms facing each other, in the regular "prayer" posture, and press the palms against each other. At the same time, lower them without letting them pull apart.

Comments

In this exercise, the real stretch is produced when you slowly lower the forearms, little by little, toward the abdomen, but without pulling the hands apart.

This is a simple exercise that can be performed at any point during the day, such as the rest periods in the middle of any long-lasting manual labor. However, it is no total substitute for the other specific exercises for stretching the fingers because it does not stretch all of them equally (the middle fingers are stretched more). This is, once again, one of the reasons why it is important to introduce variety into your training program.

 The finger flexors are muscles that are much stronger than the extensors. It could not be any other way since it is necessary to generate more force in order to grab something than to release it. However, the strength of a muscle is not reason enough to give it more or less priority when it comes to stretching. In the case of the forearms and hands, the two groups should receive the necessary mobility exercises.

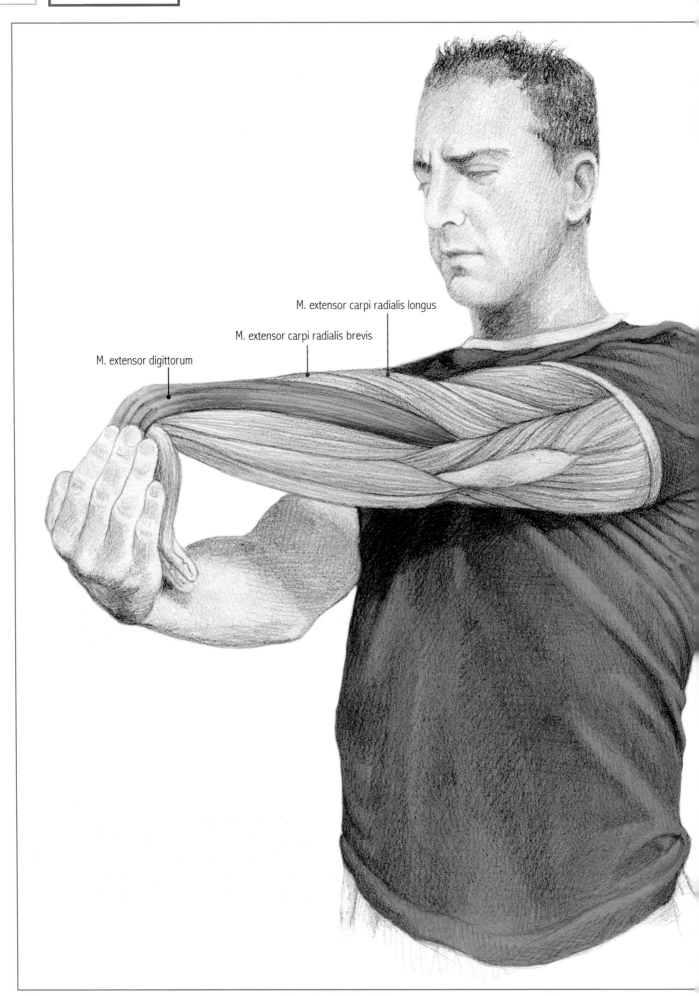

M. extensor carpi radialis longus

M. extensor carpi radialis brevis

M. extensor digittorum

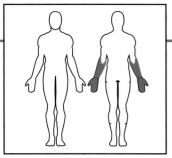

Muscles involved

Principal: Extensors of the fingers

Secondary: Extensor carpi longus and brevis

Execution

Either standing up or sitting down, extend the elbow completely at the same time that you strongly flex the wrist. The arm should remain along the length of the body.

Comments

This is a simple exercise to stretch the set of wrist and finger extensors, which can be done at any time since it does not require adopting a specific position; It can be done, for example, during your breaks from working on the computer, where the muscles that are being stretched here, normally tend to be overworked.

Another point about the stretch involves the medial rotation of the arm and forearm; that is, rotate them so that the fingers are pointing out to the sides.

 In order to understand the importance of whether or not to flex the fingers during the execution of exercises explained in this chapter, carry out this simple test: place the wrist in a natural position (in extension of the forearm, like it is when it is relaxed) and close the fist strongly; you will not have any difficulty in doing so. Now open the hand again, completely flex the wrist and once again try to make a fist. Statistically, with the hand closed the wrist will just barely exceed 75 degrees of flexion, whereas if it is open, it can reach 85 or 90 degrees.

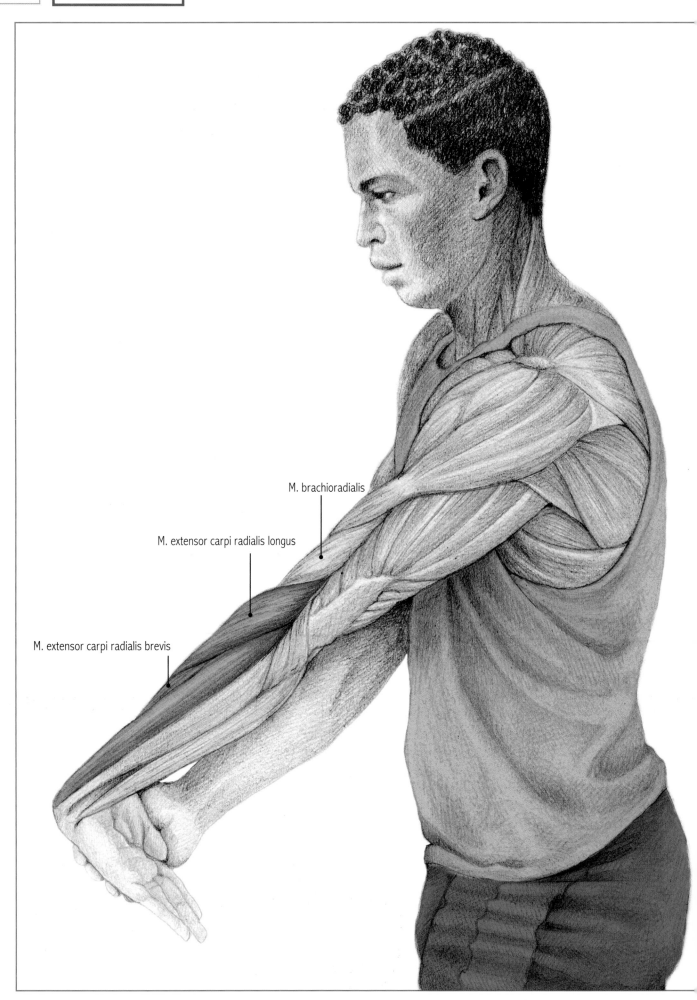

M. brachioradialis

M. extensor carpi radialis longus

M. extensor carpi radialis brevis

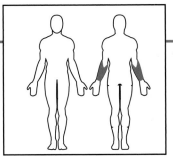

Muscles involved

Principal: Extensors of the fingers, radialis longus and brevis

Secondary: Extensor carpi longus and brevis, brachioradialis

Execution

Either standing up or sitting down, place the arm to the front with the elbow completely extended, flex the wrist and help with the other hand in order to complete the motion of this joint.

Comments

This is not a complicated exercise, which is added to the repertoire of this set of movements of the wrist, where we place special emphasis on the radial muscles.

Maintaining the elbow extended is essential in order to stretch the two-joint muscles, which cross the elbow and the wrist.

Variations

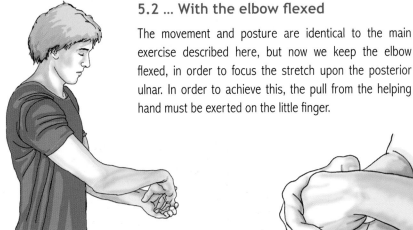

5.2 ... With the elbow flexed

The movement and posture are identical to the main exercise described here, but now we keep the elbow flexed, in order to focus the stretch upon the posterior ulnar. In order to achieve this, the pull from the helping hand must be exerted on the little finger.

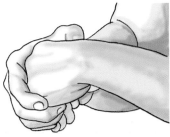

5.3 ... With the fist closed

If the exercise before had been done with the hand closed, there would have been greater tension placed upon the extensors of the fingers, without detracting from the muscles mentioned above.

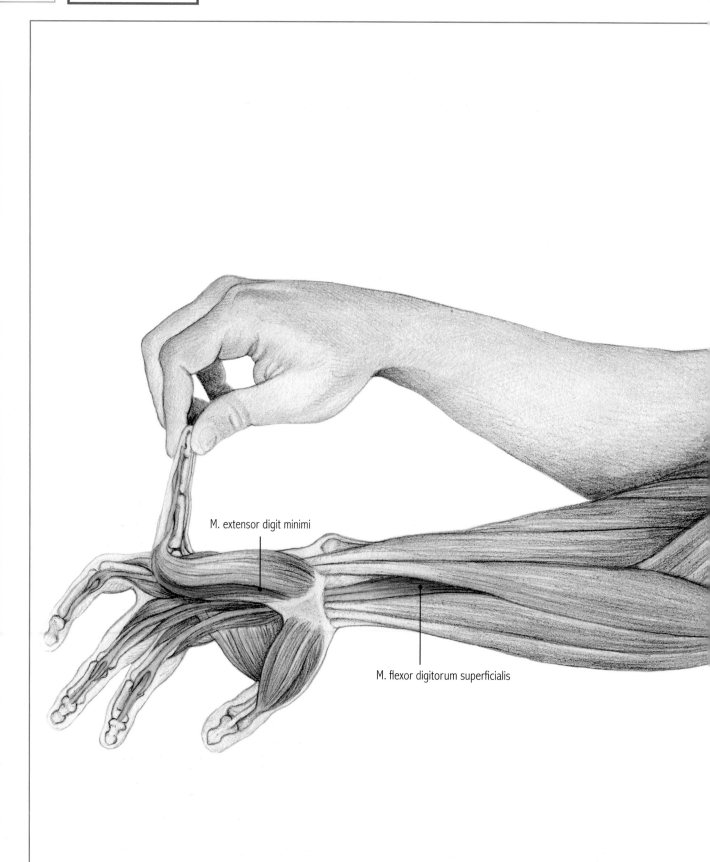

M. extensor digit minimi

M. flexor digitorum superficialis

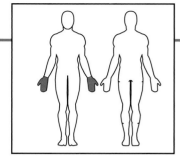

Muscles involved

Principal: The flexor muscle corresponding to the finger being extended

Execution

This simple exercise is performed by holding one finger with the other hand, and extending it individually. The stretch is maintained for a few seconds, and then one moves on to the next finger.

Comments

Even though this is a simple exercise, the pulling movement must be slow and sustained because it is not hard to injure a structure if it is done otherwise.

Some people view the stretching of each finger individually as a waste of time, feeling that it is enough to do them all together at the same time. This is a mistake, however, since there is nothing more effective than dividing up the body areas as much as possible in order to obtain the best results from stretching. The compound exercises are necessary, but the specific exercises are the true protagonists of the increases in flexibility of a specific muscle (in this case, each one of the finger extensors). The idea is much better understood by thinking about the following: a joint will only stretch as much as the worst of its muscles. In contrast to strength training, where different muscles can support one another, here the weakest link (or better yet, the stiffest) is the one that sets the pace and limits.

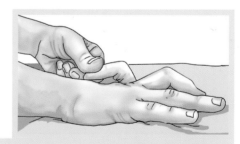

 Some people, particularly women, can extend the fingers until they touch the back of the wrist. This is know as Hypermobility Syndrome, and in most cases it is benign. However, it should not be taken lightly and anyone who has it should consult with their physician in order to confirm that it does not pose any problem, especially having ruled out the possibility of Marfan Syndrome, Ehlers-Danlos Syndrome or other uncommon pathologies. In any case, be careful to avoid some of the possible painful consequences of this particular condition (dislocations, fibromyalgia, arthritis and chondromalacia patellae, also known as CMP, Patellofemoral Pain Syndrome and Runner's Knee.

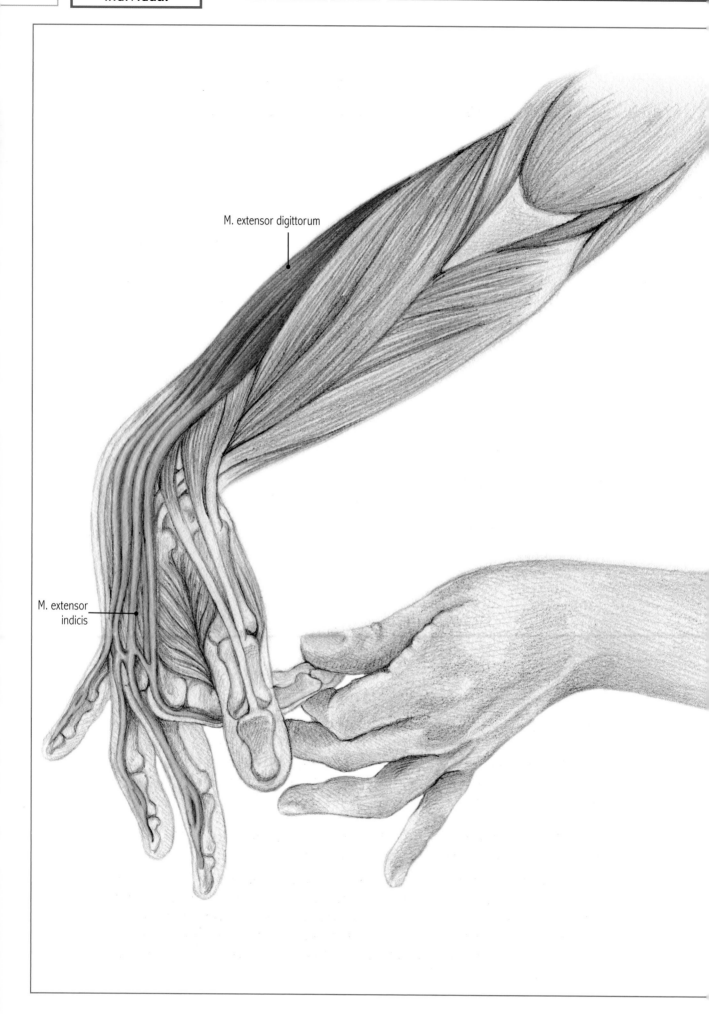

M. extensor digittorum

M. extensor indicis

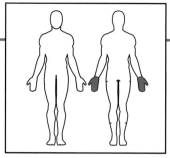

Muscles involved

Principal: The extensor muscle corresponding to the finger being flexed

Execution

Just as with the previous exercise, this one is done one finger at a time. One simply has to hold on to each finger individually with the opposite hand and produce a deep but gentle flexion. The wrist must remain flexed at approximately 90°.

Comments

In this exercise, the wrist should be flexed slightly with each pull of the finger, in order to put even greater emphasis on the tension. Of course, as in other cases, the movement here also should be slow and controlled.

Review what was mentioned about the stretching of the individual body parts in the previous segment (see exercise 6).

 There are many theories about why some joints crack when they are manipulated, particularly the joints of the fingers. Some point to the snapping of the tendons or ligaments when they are relocated, others indicate the repositioning of the joints that were slightly deviated and the subsequent crash of the joint endings (which would explain the relief that is normally felt when doing it, but not why the cracking occurs when you pull the finger, for example). Another theory mentions the unsticking of the synovial membrane that was previously adhered. The most recent theory states that, upon doing it, there is a release of the gases formed in the joint, and this is precisely what causes the cracking noises. All these different theories are not mutually exclusive, since there could be different reasons for the noises in different cases.

With respect to the dilemma about whether cracking is beneficial, harmful, or neither, there are also several contradictory theories and little scientific evidence. Some say that it corrodes the joints, whereas others say that to position them in their correct alignment is more adequate and less injurious. What is true is that it is a technique that is routinely used in physiotherapy, and that it really does achieve greater mobility and alleviates the pain when it is performed. Thus it seems unlikely that, when it is done properly and in moderation, it could be harmful.

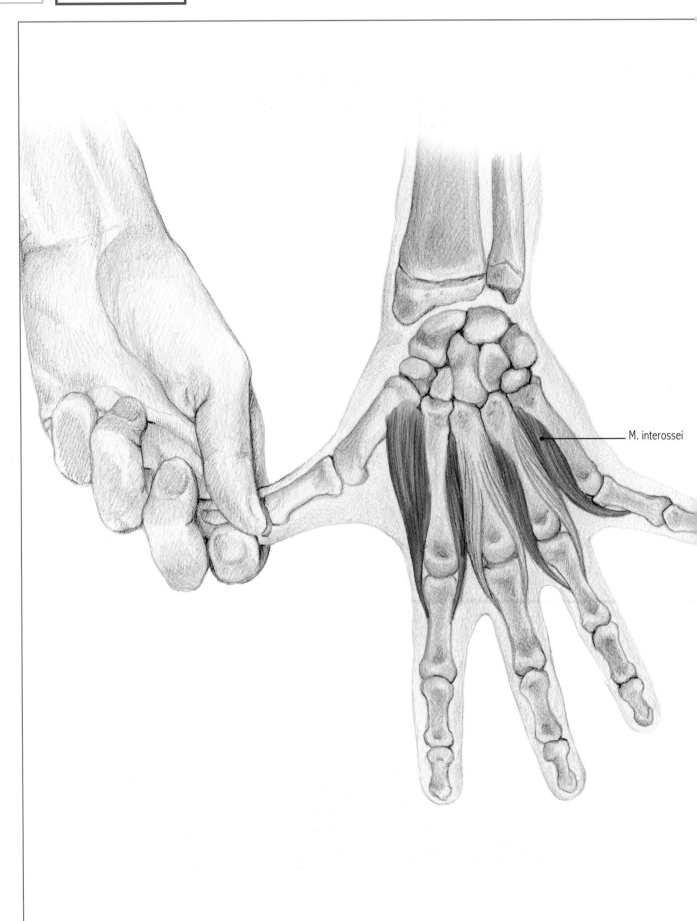

M. interossei

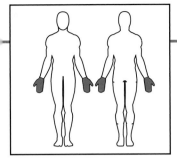

Muscles involved

Principal: Palmar interosseous, dorsal interosseous of the thumb

Secondary: Transverse ligaments of the hand

Execution

With the help of the opposite hand, the fingers are separated from each other, one by one.

Comments

Although the easiest one to separate may be the thumb (there is a reason why it is called the opposing finger), the work should involve the entire hand.

An alternative is to place an object (for example, a cylinder or a rubber ball) between the fingers and press it using the other hand toward the interdigital spaces (toward the origin of each finger). Some small muscles of the hand, such as the palmar interosseous, respond very well to this alternative.

Some professions and hobbies demand excellent finger mobility. For example, musicians who play any one of several instruments (piano, guitar, flute, etc.), will all benefit from this exercise, which they should practice conscientiously.

 The thumbs are the only fingers of the hand that are able to oppose the rest, and that is why (due to its ability to grasp) they are considered the most important for human beings, so much so that on the evolution scale, man is the most advanced and most precise. The opposition of the thumbs and bipedalism are two of the most notable human characteristics within the animal kingdom.

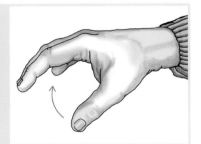

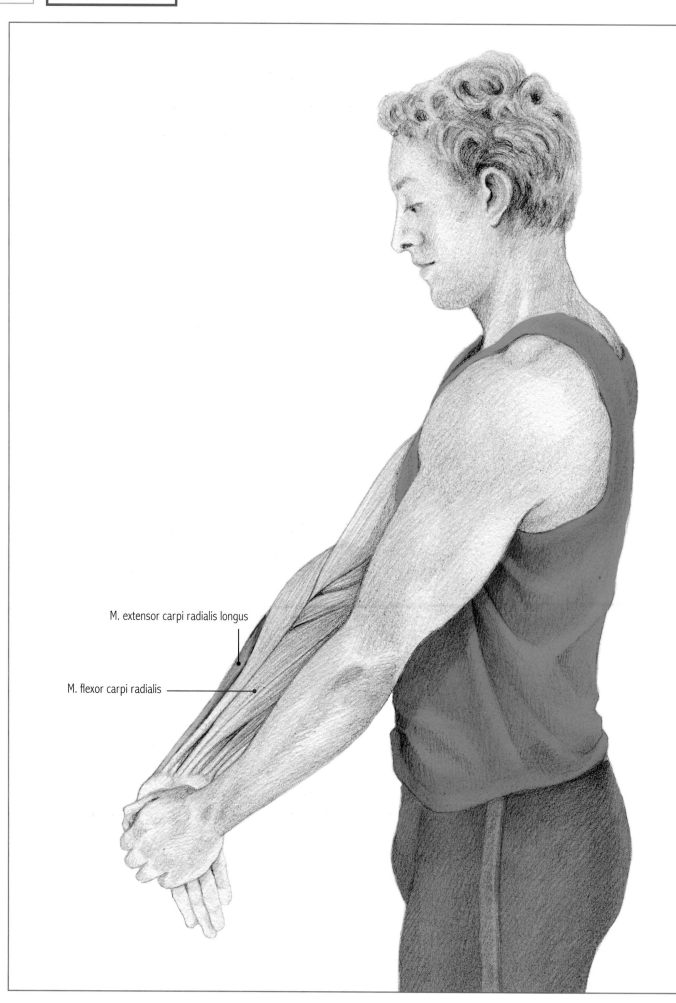

M. extensor carpi radialis longus

M. flexor carpi radialis

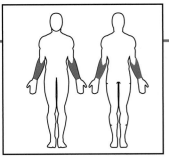

Muscles involved

Principal: Extensor carpi radialis longus, abducens policis

Secondary: Extensor policis longus, flexor carpi radialis, flexor policis longus

Execution

Begin from a starting position, preferably standing up, in which the elbow is extended completely and the hand is adducted (the little finger is brought closer toward the forearm), helping ourselves with the opposite hand, which presses on the area of the thumb.

Comments

It is important to keep the elbow extended in order to work all of the muscles indicated, otherwise we would be focusing too exclusively on the muscles of the fingers. We should not forget that some of the muscles that are stretched in this exercise are bi-jointed, meaning they cross both the elbow and the wrist.

One should not obsess about the lack of mobility of the wrist, since when it comes to abduction and adduction, it is particularly stiff. This is due more to the bony structures than to the muscles involved.

 If one is sedentary and intends to "get in shape," one first has to develop the strength, then add the flexibility exercises. Although it depends on each individual person, two months of exercise should be enough time to then add this second type of exercise.

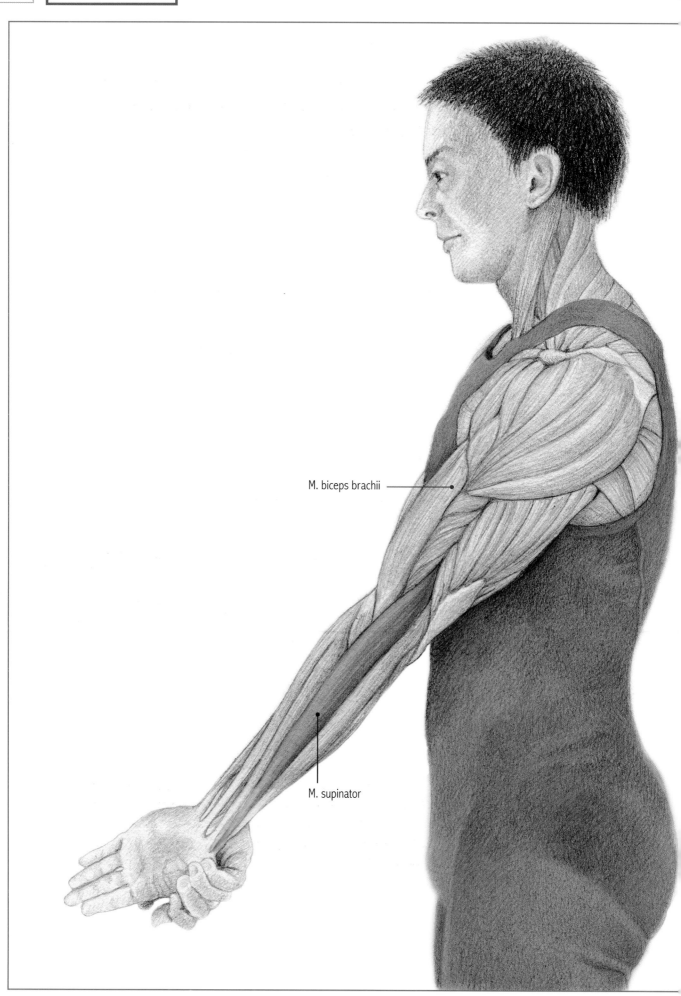

M. biceps brachii

M. supinator

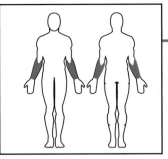

Muscles involved

Principal: Supinator, abducens policis longus, extensor policis longus

Secondary: Biceps brachii

Execution

As with the previous exercise, we begin from a starting position, preferably standing up, in which the elbow is extended completely, the hand is pronated (it is turned as if pouring a pitcher of water), helping the movement with the opposite hand.

Comments

It is not easy to stretch the muscles that are indicated here because the bony limits usually prevent it. In order to achieve this, these two movements need to be combined in order to take the muscles to their maximum extension, always maintaining the logical precautions of gentleness and no pain.

It is important to point out that pronation and supination of the forearm are not generated by the wrist, although it may look like it. The wrist, in fact, lacks those two movements. The rotation is produced at the level of the elbow, and it involves muscles of both the arm and the forearm.

 The exercises of abduction and adduction of the wrist can be practiced in the following way. Straddle a bench and place the back of the forearm and hand on top of the bench (supinated). With the other hand (and always using soft and controlled movements), proceed to the lateral turns of the hand resting on the bench. In this case, with the elbow remaining flexed, you only effectively stretch the small muscles of the wrist, not so much the ones that reach the elbow.

6

Legs Group

Descriptive anatomy of the leg: biomechanical introduction to the principal muscles

Muscles of the thigh and hip

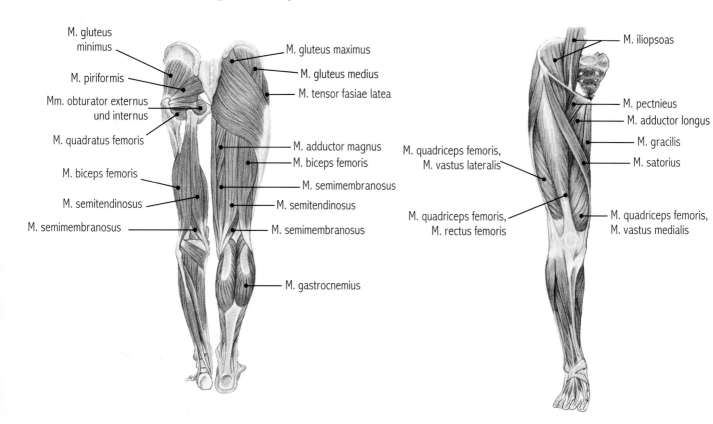

M. gluteus minimus
M. piriformis
Mm. obturator externus und internus
M. quadratus femoris
M. biceps femoris
M. semitendinosus
M. semimembranosus

M. gluteus maximus
M. gluteus medius
M. tensor fasiae latea
M. adductor magnus
M. biceps femoris
M. semimembranosus
M. semitendinosus
M. semimembranosus
M. gastrocnemius

M. iliopsoas
M. pectnieus
M. adductor longus
M. gracilis
M. satorius
M. quadriceps femoris, M. vastus lateralis
M. quadriceps femoris, M. rectus femoris
M. quadriceps femoris, M. vastus medialis

Quadriceps (anterior, superficial)

Origin: Illeum (the rectus femoris with its straight head in the anterior-inferior illiac spine; reflects it in the supra-acetabular sulcus) and femur (the vastus intermedius in the anterior and lateral surfaces, the vastus medialis in the medial labium of the linea aspera; the vastus lateralis on the lateral aspect of the greater trochanter, the intertrochanteric line, the gluteal tuberosity and the lateral labium of the linea aspera)

Insertion: Tibia (on its anterior tuberosity) and kneecap

Principal functions: Extension of the knee, the rectus femoris also strongly flexes the hip (particularly with the knee flexed). The vastus muscles also move the knee cap to their respective sides

Brachioradialis / long "supinator" (lateral, superficial)

Origin: Humerus (lateral suprachondylar border) and intermuscular septum

Insertion: Radius (external surface of the stylous process)

Principal functions: Flexion of the elbow (particularly in a neutral and pronated position) and returns the forearm to a neutral position from pronation or supination

Sartorius (anterior, superficial)

Origin: Illeum (anterior superior illiac spine)

Insertion: Tibia (medial surface, superficial pes anserinus) and crural fas

Principal functions: Assists with the flexion of the knee (exceptiona with extension, depending on the individual), as well as in the med rotation of the leg when the knee is flexed; flexion and lateral rotati of the hip

Adductors: Magnus, longus, brevis and minimus (medial, superficial and deep)

Origin: Pubis (inferior branch for the adductor magnus, brevis and minim superior branch for the adductor longus), ischium (adductor magnus)

Insertion: Femur (adductor magnus, brevis, longus, and minimus the linea aspera; adductor magnus also inserts on the adducto tubercle of the epicondyle)

Principal functions: Adduction of the thigh, secondarily also latera rotate and flex the thigh (but they can be extensors after a certa degree); adductor magnus also extends the hip. If the leg is fixed th produce anteversion (1st fascia of adductor magnus and brevis) retroversion (3rd fascia of adductor magnus)

luteus: Maximus, medius, minimus (posterior, superficial and deep)

Origin: G. Maximus originates superficially on the illiac crest and the iliac spine, the thoracolumbar fascia, the sacrum and the coccyx, and it originates deep in the illeum (from its wing) and the posterior sacrotuberal ligament. G. Medius originates in the illeum (from its wing, crest and fascia). G. Minimus originates in the illeum (gluteal surface)

Insertion: Femur (G. Maximus in the gluteal tuberosity, G. Medius and G. Minimus in the greater trochanter)

Principal functions: G. Maximus principally produces extension and external rotation of the hip, adduction and abduction (the latter by means of some of its upper fibers). G. Medus and G. Minimus (especially the first) abduction and, secondarily, medial rotation and flexion (particularly G. Minimus) or lateral rotation and extension (particularly G. Medius) according to the action of the anterior and posterior fibers, respectively

Illipsoas (anterior, deep)

Origin: Psoas major in vertebrae (lateral aspects of T12 and L1 to L4 or L5) and their corresponding intervertebral discs; psoas minor in lumbar vertebrae (lateral processes of L1 to L5). Illiopsoas in the illiac fossa (and the region of the inferior illiac spine) and adjacent ligaments

Insertion: Femur (lesser trochanter)

Principal functions: Flexion of the thigh, flexion of the trunk, internal rotation (debatable, in any case less so in flexion) and possibly adduction (many authors label it as a lateral rotator, but that is also debatable). Secondarily, lateral leaning / inclination of the trunk

Brief comments: To treat the legs as a single muscle group implies certain difficulties, since technically they do not consist of one group of muscles, just like the trunk is not composed of just a single muscle group.

There are a great number of stretching exercises for the muscles of the legs. Here, due to their fragile nature, we will emphasize the adductor muscles. It is easy to stretch them, but taking the movement to its limits is a dangerous way of getting close to their points of injury. Furthermore, in our daily lives, we do not stretch these muscles routinely. The movements in which we have to separate the legs a lot are not frequently encountered (it doesn't happen when we walk, run, sit, lay down, or in almost any daily activity).

The quadriceps and the glutes are a different story, being much more comfortable and safe to stretch. The illiopsoas deserves a special mention, being a decisive muscle in the majority of sports, but also in dance and yoga. It is one of the principal muscles responsible for the flexion of the hip (kicking the ball in soccer, running, martial arts, etc.) while at the same time, it is also a stabilizer (or a destabilizer, if it is injured in some way) of the lumbar column and the hip.

Ischiotibial: biceps femoris, semitendinosus, semimembranosus (posterior, superficial)

Origin: Long head of the bíceps, semitendinosus and semimembranosus (when it exists) in the ischium (ischial tuberosity), short head of the biceps (when it exists) in the femur (linea aspera and lateral intermuscular septum)

Insertion: Fibula (the biceps, on its external surface); tibia (semitendinosus on the superficial pes anserinus; semimembranosus, in the deep pes anserinus and on the medial condyle; the biceps on the external tibial condyle); the knee cap (with the semimembranosus forming – if it exists – the oblique popliteal ligament)

Principal functions: Extension of the hip (long head of the biceps, semimembranosus and semitendinosus; especially with the knee flexed), flexion of the knee (both heads of the biceps, semimembranosus and semitendinosus); lateral rotation of the knee (both heads of the biceps) and the hip (long head of the biceps); medial rotation of the knee and hip (semimembranosus and semitendinosus; the latter especially). If the foot is fixed, they contribute to the extension of the knee along with the gastrocnemius, and they participate in the proprioceptive function of the stability of the knee

Others

Obturator externus: Obturator foramen to the femur. Stabilizer the hip, lateral rotation, flexion and abduction of the hip

Obturator internus: Coccyx to the femur. Stabilizer of the hip, stro lateral rotation, flexion and abduction of the hip

Gracilis: Pubic bone to the tibia. Adduction of the hip; weak flex and internal rotation of the knee. Can assist in flexion and inter rotation of the hip

Pectineus: Pubic bone to the area surrounding the femur. Flex of the hip (anteversion) and weak adduction and medial rotation lateral, according to different studies or particular cases of insertio

Quadratus femoris: Ischial tuberosity to the femur. External rotatio adduction and extension (or flexion, depending on the degree)

Tensor fascia lata: Illiac spine to the tibia. Abduction and me rotation, flexion of the hip

Piriformis: Sacrum to the femur. Lateral rotation and abducti secondarily, extension (depending on degree)

Superior and inferior gemelli: Sciatic spine and ischial tuberosity the femur. Lateral rotation

Brief comments: To talk about the stretching of all the little muscles of the hip and the leg is beyond the scope of this book. But we do have to make special mention of the ischiotibial muscles. Everyone is familiar with the stretching sensation on the back of the thigh when one tries to touch the ground from a standing position, wihout bending the knees. In fact, when one wishes to demonstrate to oneself or to others, his or her degree of flexibility, this is one of the most common exercises chosen.

The ischiotibial muscles are among the muscles negatively affected by a sedentary lifestyle, as far as flexibility is concerned. Also, many athletic activities in which this area is not routinely stretched do not contribute to improving its mobility. Therefore, we can even find professional athletes who have very little flexibility in the ischiotibial muscles, despite their importance. Stretching them is extremely easy, and in this book you will find many different ways to do so.

Descriptive anatomy of the leg:
biomechanical introduction to the principal muscles

— Muscles of the leg and foot —

Tibialis anterior (anterior, superficial)

Origin: Tibia (condyle and lateral surface), interosseus membrane and crural fascia

Insertion: Medial cuneiform (plantar aspect) and first metatarsal (at its base)

Principal functions: Dorsal flexion of the foot, supination, adduction

Extensor hallucis longus (anterior, deep)

Origin: Fibula (medial surface) and interosseous membrane

Insertion: Big toe (distal phalanges) and in some people, the first metatarsal

Principal functions: Dorsal flexion of the big toe (especially the first phalanges), dorsal flexion of the foot; weak contribution to pronation and supination, depending on the position of the foot

Extensor digitorum longus (anterior, medial)

Origin: Tibia (lateral condyle), fibula (head and anterior border), crural fascia and interosseous membrane

Insertion: 2nd to 5th toes (on their dorsal aponeuroses)

Principal functions: Dorsal flexion of the foot (with a component of pronation) and extension of the toes

Others

Extensor digitorum brevis: Calcaneous to the first 4 toes. Extension (dorsal flexion) of those toes

Extensor hallucis brevis: Calcaneous to the big toe. Dorsal flexion of the big toe

Dorsal interosseous: Between the 5 toes. Separates them from each other

Plantar interosseous: From the last 3 metatarsals to the 1st phalanges of last 3 toes. Brings toes together

Lumbrical muscles: Between the toes. Flex the first phalanges and extend the other two

Quadratus plantaris: Calcaneous to the tendon of flexor digitorum longus. Complements and corrects said flexor muscle

Brief comments: The best way to stretch this area is either sitting or lying down. They are not impressive muscles (although no less important) but they are mistreated by today`s way of life. Everyone can understand that man has gone from walking barefoot to walking with shoes, from moving about by walking or running to doing so using transportation; and that these changes have meant countless advantages. But the small muscles of the foot have been adversely affected by these changes. Many types of shoes compress and immobilize the toes and the ankles, resulting in their atrophy and deformation. Their strengthening (see "Encyclopedia of Bodybuilding Excercises" Ed. Pila Teleña) and their stretching are vital for their well-being.

Gastrocnemius (posterior, superficial)

Origin: Femur (medial and lateral heads of the femoral condyles), joint capsule of the knee (part of its fasciculi)

Insertion: Calcaneous (posterior tuberosity)

Principal functions: Plantar flexion of the foot (especially with the knee extended), flexion of the knee, supination of the foot. With the foot fixed, it collaborates, together with the ischiotibial muscles, in the extension of the knee

Soleus (posterior, medial)

Origin: Fibula (head and upper and dorsal neck of the same), tibia (soleus line) and tendinous arch of the soleus (between the head of the fibula and tibia)

Insertion: Calcaneous (posterior tuberosity)

Principal functions: Plantar flexion of the foot (in a more isolated manner with the knee flexed), flexion of the knee, supination of the foot

Others

Peroneus: Long and short. Fibula to the first metatarsal and cuneiform (long) and fifth metatarsal (short). Maintaining the plantar arch, strong pronation, plantar flexion

Popliteal: Femur to the tibia. Flexion of the knee (or extension according to other authors) and medial rotation of the leg, "active ligament" of the knee

Tibialis posterior: Tibia, fibula, and interosseous membrane to Navicular and 3 cuneiform of the foot (plantar aspect). Plantar flexion, adduction, supination and maintenance of the plantar arch

Plantaris: Femur to Achilles tendon. Plantar flexion of the foot

Flexor hallucis longus: Fibula, interosseous membrane and posterior intermuscular septum to distal phalanges of the big toe. Flexion of the big toe, plantar flexion, adduction and supination of the foot, and maintenance of the plantar arch

Flexor digitorum longus: Tibia to terminal phalanges of toes 2 to 5. Flexion of said toes, and plantar flexion, adduction and supination of the foot, and maintenance of the plantar arch

Flexor digitorum brevis: Calcaneus to toes 2 to 5. Flexion of the 2nd phalanges of said toes over the 1st

Flexor hallucis brevis: 2nd and 3rd cuneiform and cuboidal, to 1st phalanges of big toe. Flexion of the 1st phalanges and extension of the 2nd

Adductor hallucis: Calcaneous to the big toe. Adducts the first phalanges, flexes and extends the 2nd

Adductor obliquus hallucis: Cuboidal, 3rd cuneiform and 3rd and 4th metatarsals to the big toe. Balances the abductor and contributes to maintaining the plantar arch

Transversus hallucis: Glenoid ligament of the 3rd, 4th and 5th metatarsophalangeal joints, to the big toe

Brief comments: People who run frequently, or who for whatever reason, get around on foot, are aware that stretching the muscles of the calf is important. Focusing the effort on one or another area will depend on the position of the feet and also of the knee. In this way, the stretches performed with the knee extended will work primarily the gastrocnemius, while those performed with the knee flexed will work primarily the soleus.

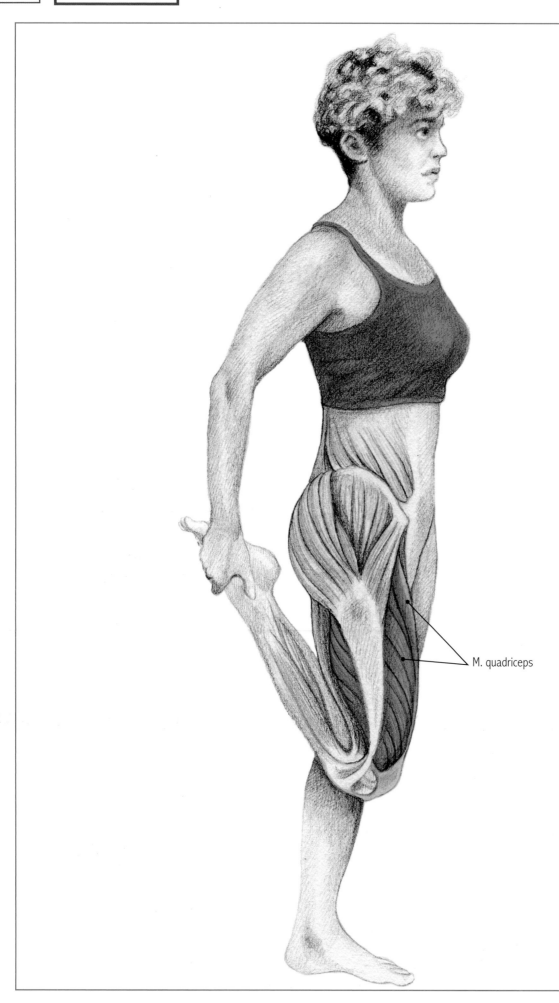

M. quadriceps

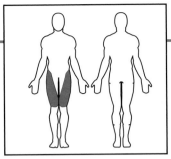

Muscles involved

Principal: Quadriceps
Secondary: Illiopsoas

Execution

Standing up, leaning against a support in order to maintain balance, flex a knee and hold on to the dorsum medial aspect of the foot that is raised using the ipsilateral hand. Press the heel of the foot against the gluteus to stretch the quadriceps.

Comments

The hip should not be flexed, nor should you lean the torso, but it is recommended to extend the hip a little bit backwards on the side that is being worked in order to get a good stretch on a portion of the quadriceps, the rectus femoris (which is bi-jointed).

If the hip moves in the opposite way (that is, raising the knee in front of the body but maintaining the rest of the posture as is) then you will be placing emphasis on the vastus lateralis and medialis of the quadriceps, taking some of the tension off the rectus femoris.

Having a support to maintain your balance is not trivial; in any stretching exercise, the lack of balance is a factor that detracts efficacy.

Variation   **1.2... Lying on your side**

If you place yourself in a lateral decubitus position (lying on your side) and you proceed to stretch in the manner that was described above, you will achieve the same effect. The advantage is avoiding the frequent lordosis and other inadequate postures of the column and the hip which tend to occur when we are standing up, at times the result of maintaining our balance on just one leg.

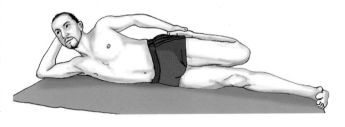

We should remember that the rectus femoris of the quadriceps is not effectively stretched with just a simple flexion of the knee, it has to be accompanied by a light extension of the hip; otherwise, one of the vastus muscles of the quadriceps will not receive an adequate stretch.

In this exercise, some people tend to cause a rotation of the knee by carrying the foot farther than the gluteus. Without a doubt, this can produce a greater stretch of the quadriceps, but it also unnecessarily forces the ligaments of the knee (see exercise 9.3).

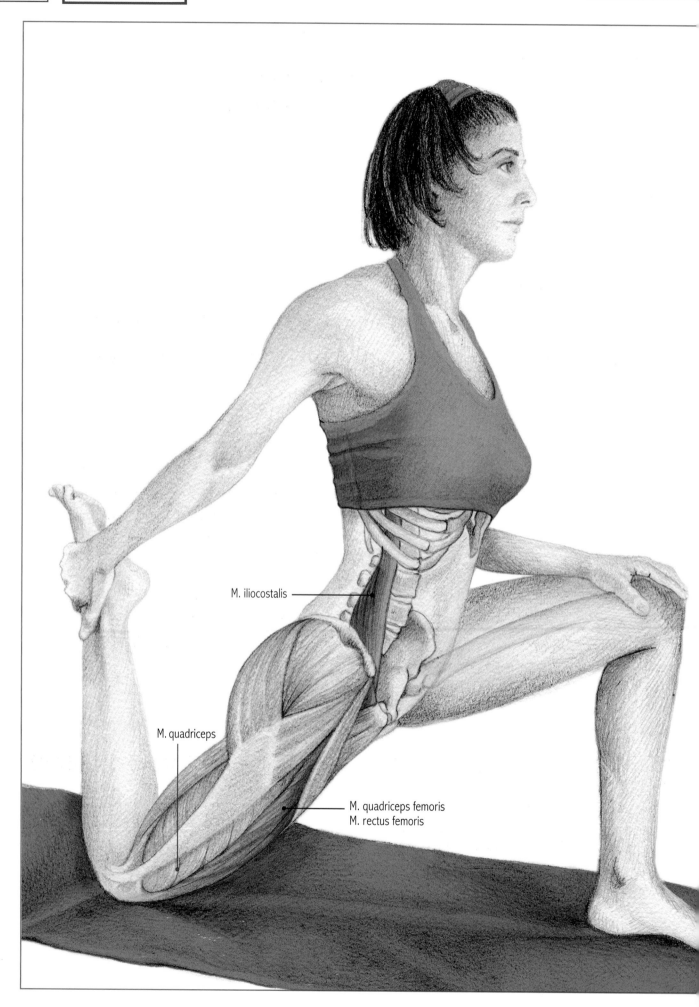

M. iliocostalis

M. quadriceps

M. quadriceps femoris
M. rectus femoris

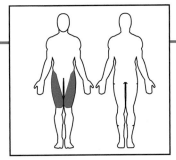

Muscles involved

Principal: Illiopsoas, rectus femoris of the quadriceps

Secondary: Quadriceps

Execution

Place a foot firmly on the padded ground, with the knee at the same level (mainly do not bring the knee farther forward than the foot that supports it), and take the other leg farther back, resting the knee on the ground. Pull on the ankle of the leg that is behind, bringing it toward the gluteus at the same time that you push the pelvis downward and forward.

Comments

This exercise is similar to the first exercise described in the chapter, but while maintaining the leg that is being stretched farther back (in extension of the hip) you also bring into play the hip flexors, especially the illiopsoas. The combination of hip extension and knee flexion makes this exercise very appropriate for stretching the quadriceps group (remember that one of its components – the rectus femoris – crosses both joints). And, on the other hand, to focus the stretch on the illiopsoas, but not so much on the quadriceps, it is enough simply to not hold on to the foot, but place it against the ground with the inside of the foot and leave the knee semi-extended at the same time that you press even more on the pelvis.

In summary, this exercise, when performed correctly, is one of the most effective for stretching the quadriceps.

Variation　　　**2.2... On a bench**

The same exercise may be performed while lying on a bench (for some people this is more comfortable). This support also allows for the entire trunk to be resting upon the bench, but that would greatly reduce the stretch of the hip flexors, and making it just a stretch for the quadriceps.

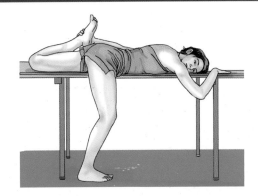

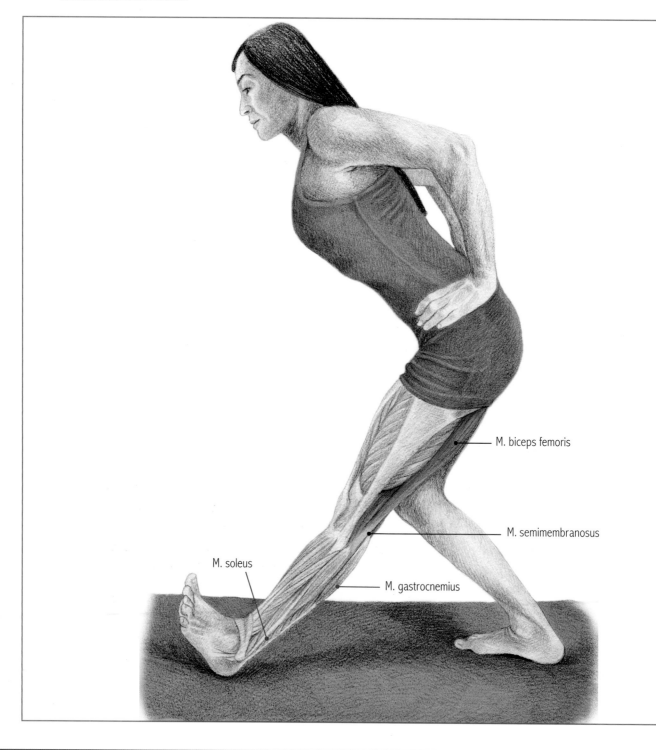

M. biceps femoris

M. semimembranosus

M. soleus

M. gastrocnemius

Variation   **3.2... Over a support**

If there is a tall enough support available (at least to the height of the waist of the person stretching), he or she can rest the heel of the foot upon it, and, with the knee extended, flex the hip slightly until he or she feels the tension on the back of the thigh; meanwhile, the foot on the ground must be pointing forward. The problem with shorter supports is that they force the person to lean over them too much in order to achieve the desired tension in the stretch, adding a component of balance that "pollutes" the exercise.

Let's not forget that the objective is not to "touch the foot" but rather to produce a sufficient stretch of the ischiotibial

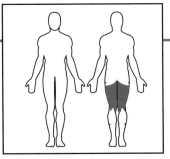

Muscles involved

Principal: Ischiotibialis

Secondary: Gracilis, sartorius, popliteal, gastrocnemius and soleus
(if the foot is dorsiflexed)

Execution

From a standing position, one leg is slightly flexed and the other is extended to the front, supporting the heel. The knee must remain perfectly extended, to favor the stretch of the ischiotibialis. The spine must remain aligned (and the head as a continuation of the spine) just like in the majority of the exercises.

Comments

This simple exercise is effective for stretching the ischiotibialis of the leg in front; it is just a little bit more complex than the traditional "touch the tip of your toes from a standing position" and much more effective. The reason why has already been explained in other parts of this book; it is not convenient that the muscle we are about to stretch is contracted in an effort to maintain our posture. Therefore, it is the leg that is pushed to the back   is the one that supports the weight, and here lies part of the difficulty in this exercise.

The variation in which we remain perfectly seated on a bench or something similar, and extend one leg on the ground to resemble the posture that is explained here, is not entirely advisable (except if it is done over a padded support), since the edge of the bench could press precisely the area that we are aiming to stretch. The most advisable position out of all these involves supporting the entire leg over the bench, making the most of its length, and leaning over it.

muscles, and the key is in the hip. In fact, to increase the tension of the stretch, it is not advisable to increase the height of the support where we place our foot, which would make balance more difficult, but rather flex the hip in such a way that we bring the torso closer to the leg that is in front.

This series of exercises for stretching the ischiotibial muscles involves a similar difficulty in execution: the person normally has the tendency to lower as far as possible and in order to do so, flexes the trunk, curves the spine, but does not actually flex the hip. Learning to feel exactly where the muscle is being stretched is imperative.

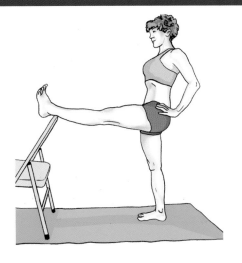

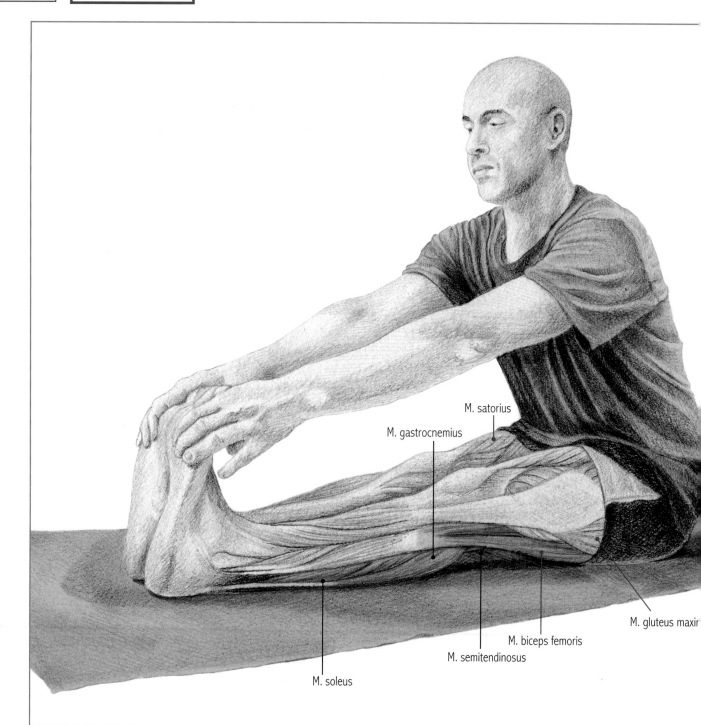

M. satorius

M. gastrocnemius

M. gluteus maxir⟩

M. biceps femoris

M. semitendinosus

M. soleus

Variations | **4.2... Standing up**

In this exercise, which can basically seem to be the same, one of the basic rules this book attempts to impart is broken; a muscle being stretched must not, at the same time, be under tension to maintain a posture. In other words, this time we are going to stretch some muscles which, in turn, we must contract to avoid losing our balance; and the results are not very satisfactory.

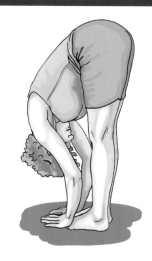

The traditional bounces to try ⟩ reach farther down only aggrav⟩ the situation, because they trigger ⟩ myotic, which causes the ischioti⟩ muscles to contract even fart⟩ Therefore, one of the most clas⟩ stretching exercises is also one of ⟩ most inappropriate.

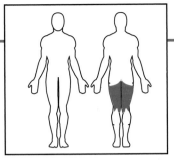

Muscles involved

Principal: Ischiotibial muscles, gastrocnemius, soleus

Secondary: Gluteus maximus, gracilis, sartorius, popliteal, tibialis posterior, peroneus, plantaris

Execution

Seated, with both legs together at the front and the knees completely extended, the hip is flexed until you feel the tension on the back of the thigh, in the ischiotibial muscles.

Comments

This exercise is similar to those explained in the previous pages. Here, however, we eliminate the bothersome component of balance that ocassionally interferes during the exercises performed standing up. The exercise is not as simple as it may seem, and the most common mistake is to flex the trunk ("curve your back"), while the correct thing to do is to perform the flexion truly at the hip. One common mistake is to flex the knees at the same time that one tries to lower oneself more, doubtlessly in order to alleviate some of the tension on the ischiotibial muscles.

Beginners will barely be able to form a right angle, while advanced individuals will be able to touch their thighs with their forehead; these people can even hold the bottom of their feet with their hands. But the objective of the exercise is not to reach as far as possible with the hands, but rather to produce a sufficient twist of the hip in order to stretch the ischiotibial muscles; confusing the objective of the exercise could lead to one of the bad postures that we have just described.

The help of a partner can be simply pushing on the middle of the back, or getting down back to back and unloading the weight upon the person doing the stretch, with the usual precautions that apply to all outside assistance.

4.3... Standing up, with legs crossed

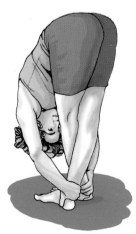

In an attempt to search for variety, although not originality, some people cross their legs and perform this exercise. The same negative comments which were made for the previous variation also apply here.

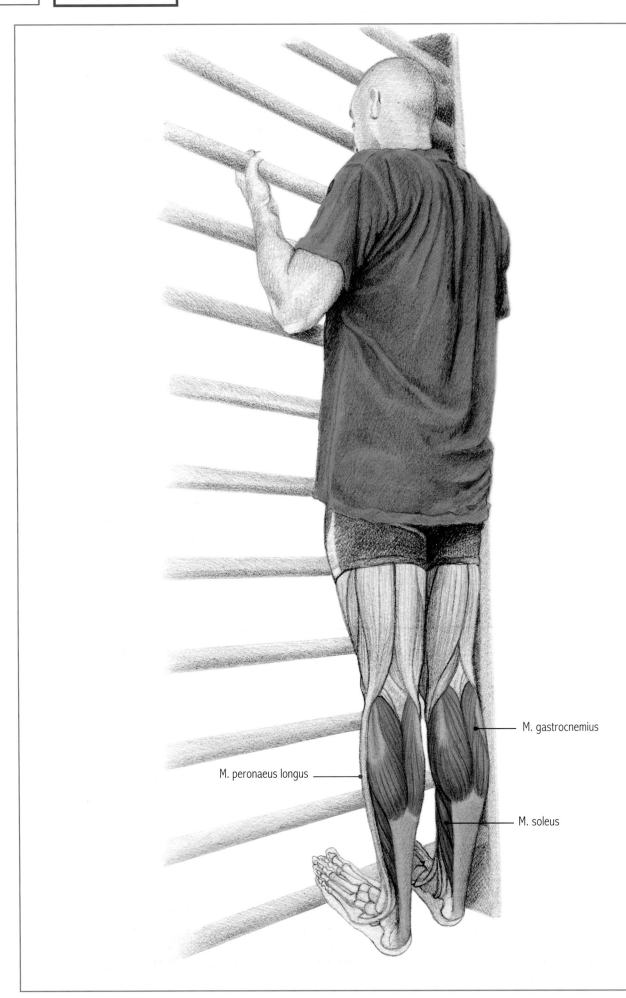

M. gastrocnemius

M. peronaeus longus

M. soleus

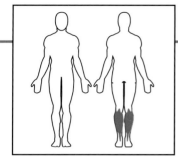

Muscles involved

Principal: Gastrocnemius, soleus

Secondary: Peroneus, flexor digitorum longus, tibialis posterior, plantaris

Execution

Standing up, with the knees extended, we place ourselves over a step (a single step, stairs, etc.), supporting only the front half of the foot. We let the body fall gently while we notice the tension in the gastrocnemius and soleus.

Comments

Better results are obtained if you gently rest (in a slow movement) the weight over the posture maintained. The knee should never flex and under no circumstances should you bounce, something that in addition to inhibiting progress, could produce injuries if the person is tired or under the right circumstances. You should also not rest only the toes upon the step, because in addition to increasing the risk of the foot falling from its support, you would not increase the stretch of the gastrocnemius or the soleus. In fact, in this exercise it is more appropriate to use athletic shoes with a good grip than to perform it barefoot.

The body weight is enough for an optimal stretch; adding extra weight could lead, once more, to an injury. If the area is very overloaded (for example, after a long race) it might be advisable to substitute this exercise for another one where the tension is more controllable (see exercise 6).

Do not let your feet turn inward or outward in an attempt to stretch the lateral external or internal zones, but rather simply perform the exercise with the feet in parallel, even though some books may recommend such turns. It appears necessary, therefore, to remember that these turns are produced at the hip, not at the knee, and so they do not affect the gastrocnemius (which, obviously, do not reach the hip). It is also not advisable in this exercise to perform the movements of eversion and inversion of the foot, being preferable to leave this for the manual manipulation that is explained in subsequent exercises in this book.

 Given that all the movements are described in an "anatomical position" (see Dictionary at the end of the book), it is a little ambiguous to talk about flexion or extension of the ankle. To avoid any such conclusions, other terms are used in this book, terms that are also correct and unequivocal: tibial flexion when the foot is brought closer to the tibia at the front (flexion), and plantar flexion when the opposite occurs (extension).

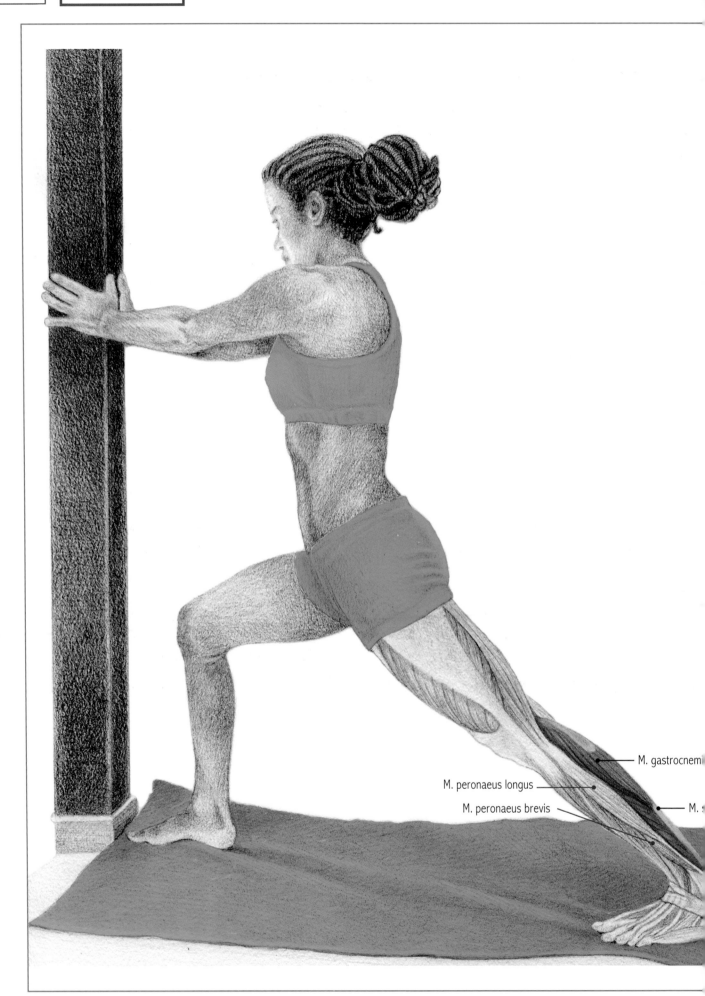

M. gastrocnem

M. peronaeus longus

M. peronaeus brevis

M.

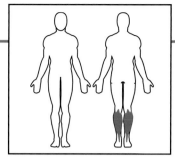

Muscles involved

Principal: Gastrocnemius, soleus

Secondary: Peroneus, flexor digitorum longus, tibialis posterior, plantaris

Execution

Standing up, holding on to a support, one leg is pushed backwards and – with the knee extended – the entire sole of the foot is rested on the ground, in such a way that the tension of the stretch is felt in the area of the gastrocnemius. The forward leg remains semi-flexed, supporting the weight of the body.

Comments

The most important thing in this exercise is to keep the knee extended, otherwise you will only be stretching the soleus. The point of maximum stretch is achived by gently placing the heel of the back leg on the ground and holding that position, and for that you will have to slowly and progressively displace the weight from the front leg to the back leg to progressively lower the heel in the manner described.

There are two techniques to adjust the degree of stretch: keep the knee extended and progressively lower the heel until it fully touches the ground and move the heel even farther to the back; or keep the heel on the floor the entire time and slowly extend the knee and the hip in order to increase the tension.

In all cases, the foot remains aligned with the knee and with the hip, with the toes pointing toward the front.

 Is it possible to nullify or deactivate the myostatic reflex? The answer is no. As is the case with every reflex, the myostatic reflex is produced unconsciously and, furthermore, it is an important reflex in terms of preventing injuries during our everyday lives and sporting activities. What one can do is prevent if from appearing with intensity during a stretch; this can be achieved by performing slow and controlled movements, although it requires training and practice.

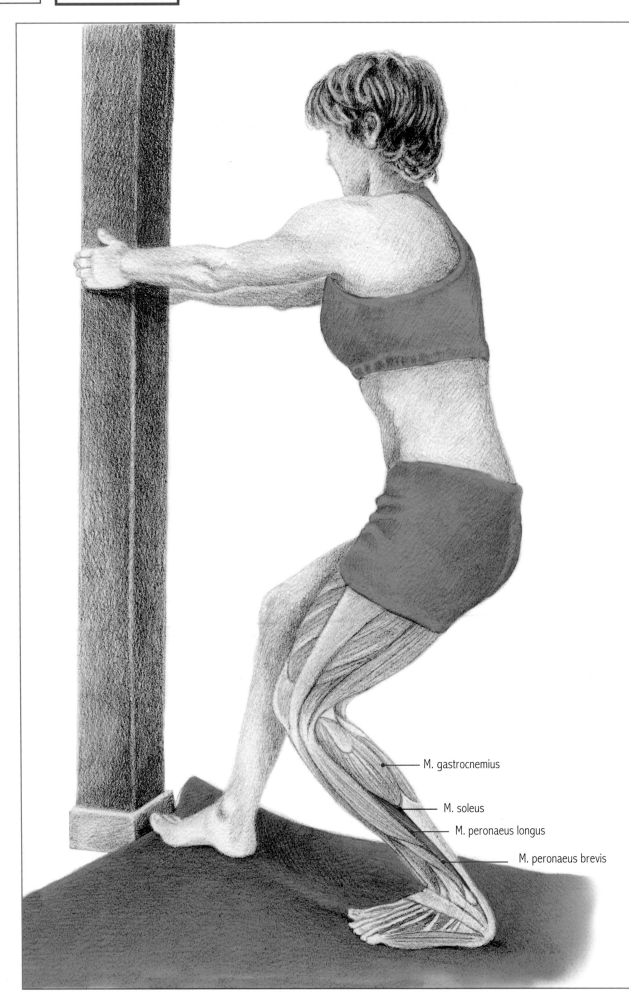

M. gastrocnemius

M. soleus

M. peronaeus longus

M. peronaeus brevis

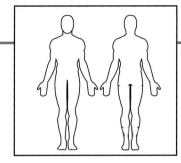

Muscles involved

Principal: Soleus

Secondary: Gastrocnemius, peroneus, tibialis posterior

Execution

Standing up, holding on to a support, one leg is pushed backward and – with the knee semiflexed – the entire sole of the foot is planted on the ground, in such a way that the tension is felt in the area of the soleus (below the gastrocnemius). The forward leg remains in semi-flexion, supporting the weight of the body.

Comments

In contrast to the previous exercise that was described, what is important during this exercise is to keep the knee in flexion, to place more emphasis on the stretching of the soleus. The point of maximum stretch is achieved, once again, by gently placing the heel of the back leg on the ground.

The most common way of adjusting the tension over the soleus is to progressively bring the knee closer to the wall without lifting the heel off the ground (in order to flex the ankle more).

This exercise with the knee bent can also be performed on a step (see exercise 5), although it can be somewhat uncomfortable.

 The more appropriate name for the tendon, which is the distal insertion point for the gastrocnemius and soleus, is the "tendon of the triceps surae," and while it is permissible to call it "Achilles' tendon," it is not acceptable to refer to it as "Achilles' heel."

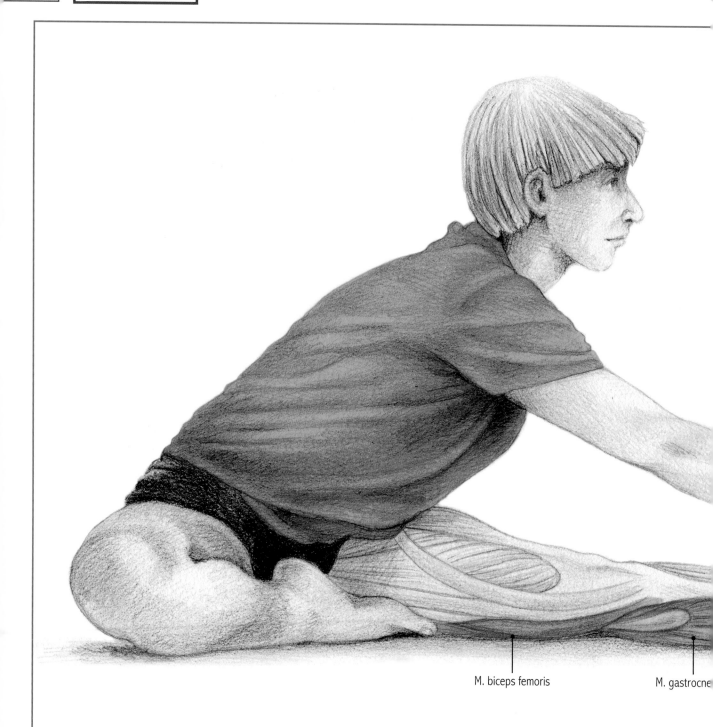

M. biceps femoris   M. gastrocne

Execution

Seated on the ground with one leg flexed over itself, that is, the knee is flexed and the heel of the foot rested upon the adductor muscles of the opposite leg. The front leg is the one being stretched, and thu it must remain with the knee extended.

From this position, the hip is flexed, lowering the trunk toward the outstretched leg.

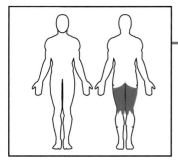

Muscles involved

Principal: Ischiotibial muscles, gastrocnemius, soleus

Secondary: Gluteus maximus, gracilis, sartorius, popliteal, adductors, tibialis posterior, peroneus, flexors of the toes, plantaris

Comments

As with other similar exercises, the spinal column and the head should remain aligned. Those people with limited flexibility tend to flex the trunk over itself, believing that they are progressing in the stretching of the ischiotibial muscles when they feel how they are getting closer to the front leg, but it should not be this way.

Why is one of the legs flexed? There is no problem with not doing it, just as it was explained in the previous pages, but in this way the stretch upon the hip flexors is reduced, since only one side is being worked.

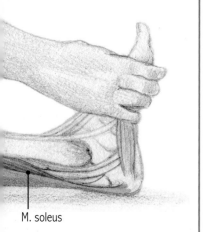

M. soleus

8.2... Variation with the opposite leg behind the back

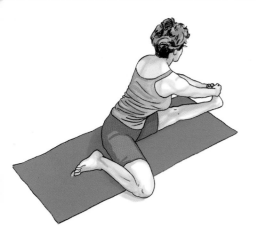

Occasionally, the person performing the stretch places the leg that is not being worked behind herself. This does not mean any changes for the principal muscles being stretched (especially the ischiotibial muscles, gastrocnemius and soleus), but it is harmful to some of the structures of the knee that is flexed, especially the ligaments. Therefore, this variation (also called "hurdler") doesn't make any sense and its widespread acceptance in the world of sports is surprising. The only acceptable exception would be in the sports-specific training of the pole vaulters, although their performance does not vary in any significant way if this exercise is substituted for others.

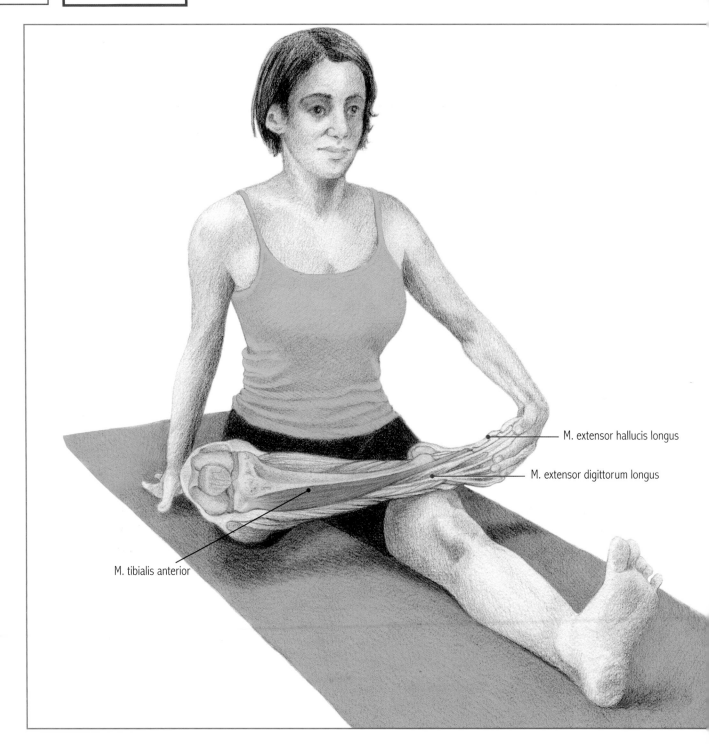

M. extensor hallucis longus

M. extensor digittorum longus

M. tibialis anterior

Variations | **9.2... Seated on the heels**

If the floor is slightly padded, the previous exercise can be done in a very simple manner, simply by sitting on top of the heels, just as is shown in the image. The entire medial aspect of the foot must be touching the ground.

In order to increase the stress on the tibial region, you may use a little extra padding – such as a folded towel – underneath the feet (but not underneath the ankles).

One last variation in which the metatarsals and the toes are supported (preferably flexed), does not stretch the tibialis, but rather the flexors of the toes (which are found in the plantar region).

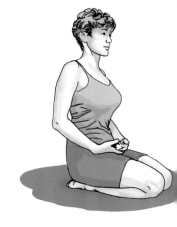

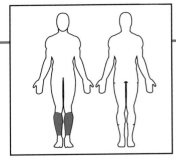

Muscles involved

Principal: Tibialis anterior

Secondary: Extensor digitorum longus and extensor hallucis longus

Execution

Seated (either on the ground or on a bench), cross one leg over the other and pull on the medial aspect of the foot in plantar flexion (that is, inward).

Comments

Stretching the tibialis anterior is extremely easy. The ideal is for the whole hand to cover the foot and the toes, in such a way that as you progressively pull toward the back, the tension is felt on the anterior part of the leg. Although this is not a very complex exercise, runners know of the importance of stretching this muscle. On occasion, people suffer from pain in the tibial area due to continued stress or inflammation of the area, and this stretch is part of the training to prevent and alleviate it.

On the other hand, if the traction is not applied covering the entire medial surface of the foot, but rather just on the toes, we will focus the stretch upon the short and long extensors of the toes (extensor digitorum brevis and extensor digitorum longus).

9.3... Seated between the feet

This is done in an almost identical way to the previous variant, but opening the legs a little bit in order to be able to sit on the ground, between the feet.

This variation is not recommended, since it unnecessarily stresses the knee joints, as you may notice that to the hyperextension component has been added a component of joint rotation. Some people with enough flexibility adopt this posture frequently (for example, veteran practitioners of yoga or dance), something which should be avoided. Just because the body is able to perform a movement or tolerate a posture does not mean that one should necessarily do it.

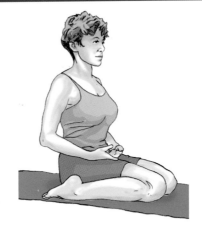

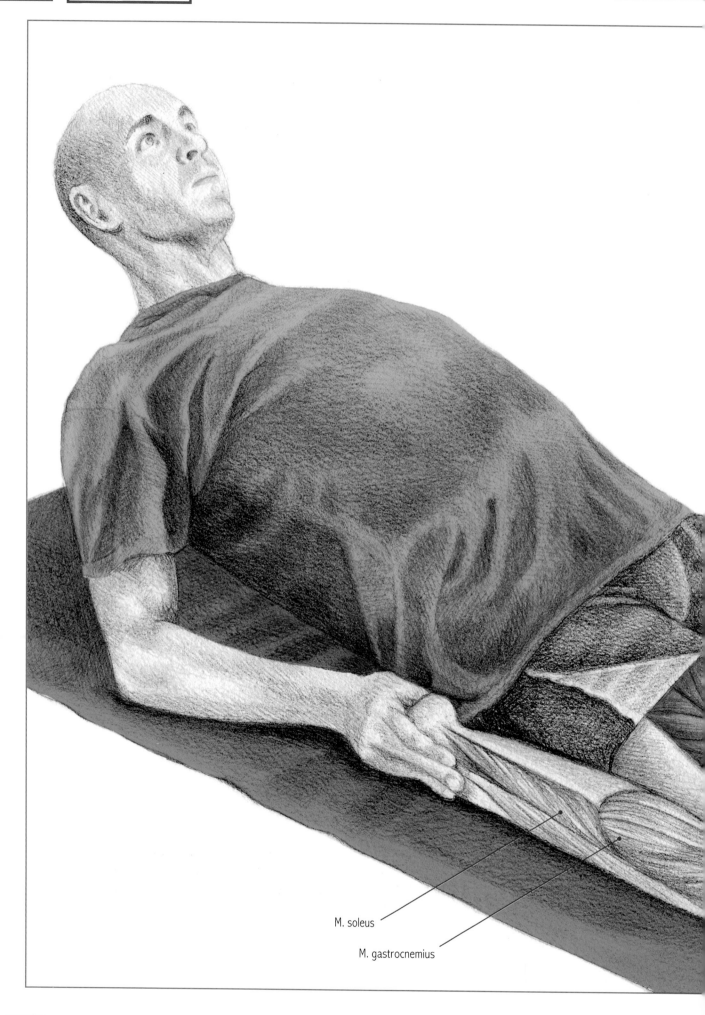

M. soleus

M. gastrocnemius

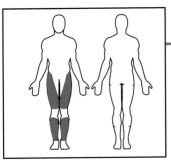

Muscles involved

Principal: Quadriceps

Secondary: Illiopsoas, tibialis anterior, extensor digitorum longus and extensor hallucis longus

Execution

Seated on top of your heels, preferably upon a padded surface, extend the hip and allow the trunk to fall backward in a controlled fashion.

Comments

This exercise is similar to the variation explained previously (see exercise 9.2), but the leaning of the body backward extends the quadriceps, which are added to the list of muscles already being worked. Because of the position that is adopted, the hip flexors also participate.

The discomfort inherent in the position makes this exercise fairly uncommon, and the muscles worked may be stretched with other more comfortable and effective exercises. Not all stretching exercises have to be comfortable (just like other physical activities, it requires a certain degree of effort), but there are some movements and activities that, in addition to being uncomfortable, are also not so effective so as to make the effort worthwhile. Athletes tend to have a greater tolerance for discomfort and physical effort than sedentary people, but one must not confuse effort with a job well done.

M. quadriceps femoris

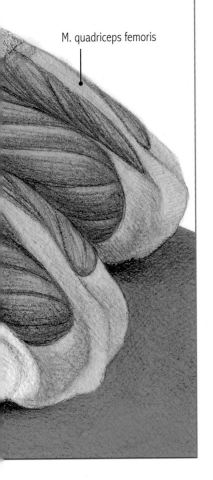

 It is not advisable to perform an intense stretching session just before an intense session of physical activity. It is safer and more advisable to perform a few light stretches between the warm-up and the physical activity itself.

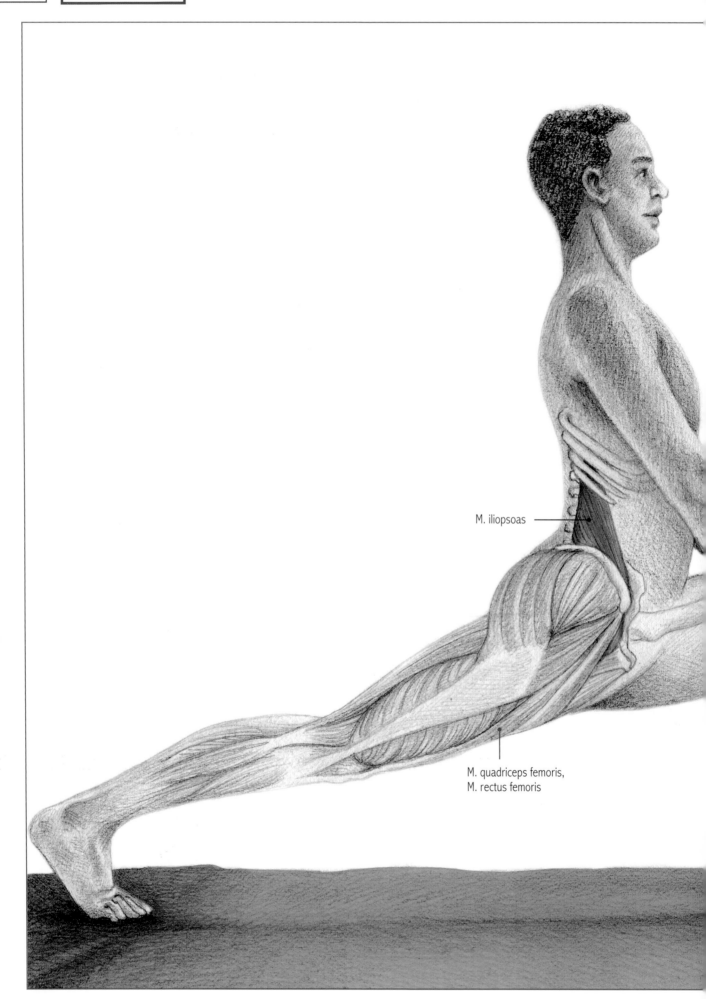

M. iliopsoas

M. quadriceps femoris,
M. rectus femoris

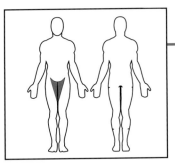

Muscles involved

Principal: illiopsoas

Secondary: Rectus femoris, adductors, pectineus, gluteus maximus

Execution

From a standing position, bring the body forward with a great stride without lifting the back foot off the ground. From this position, flex the back knee and the majority of the bodyweight is now supported by the front leg. The front knee must remain right above the foot, and should never go beyond the foot. Lower the weight of the trunk vertically (bring the pelvis toward the floor) to increase the stretch.

Comments

With this simple and extended exercise, we especially work the hip flexors. To keep your balance, you can rest your hands on the front leg or a side bench, this support is vitally important in order to be able to perform this exercise correctly.

If you had to choose only one exercise to stretch the illiopsoas, this would be it, because of its simplicity and effectiveness. There is a variation in which you do not support the metatarsals of the foot, but rather its medial surface, and this implies a change in the muscles being stretched, which in this case primarily means adding the tibialis anterior and the anterior ulnar to the list.

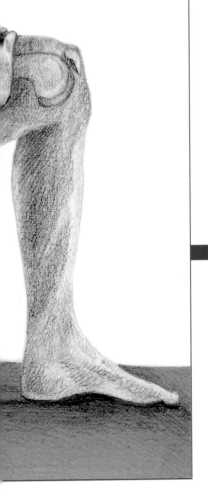

Variation

11.2... On a bench

The exercise is basically the same, but now the front leg is rested on top of a raised support. The differences in the muscles worked are minimal, although the author continues to prefer the previous exercise.

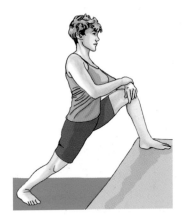

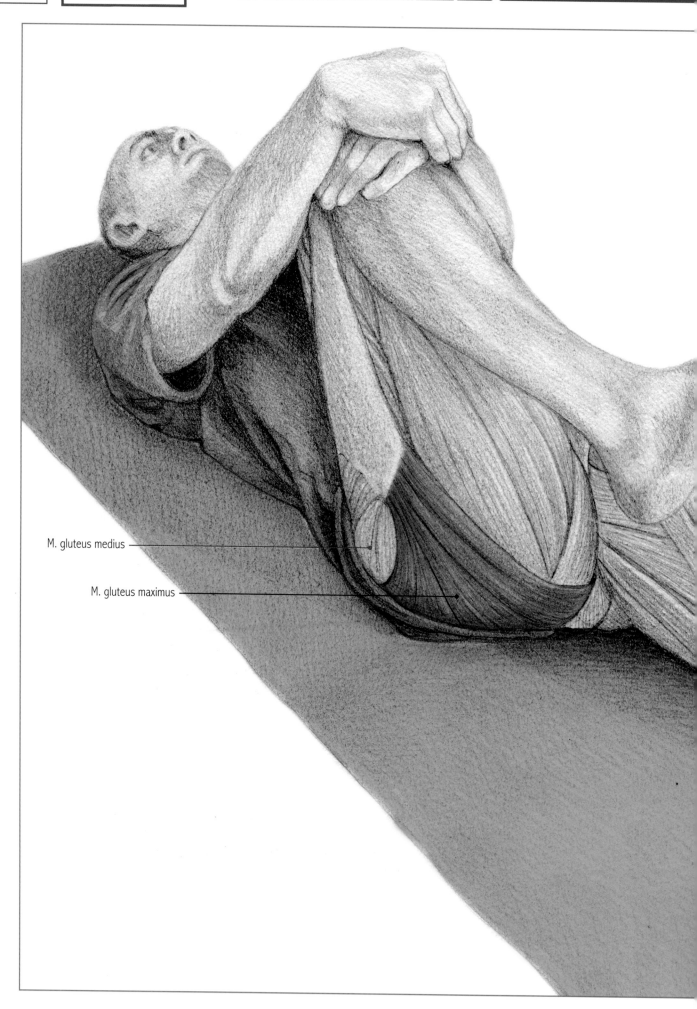

M. gluteus medius

M. gluteus maximus

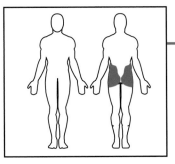

Muscles involved

Principal: Gluteus maximus

Secondary: Gluteus medius and minimus (of the extended leg: illiopsoas)

Execution

Lying on the ground, one leg is flexed (both at the hip and at the knee) and "hugged" with both hands, pressing the leg against the chest. The other leg remains extended on the ground.

Comments

This simple exercise stretches the gluteus of the elevated leg, but secondarily, the hip flexors of the extended leg are also stretched. People with a low degree of flexibility will notice how the leg, which should remain on the ground, naturally lifts up, something they should avoid (for example, by placing the foot under a bar).

In this exercise, the help of a partner could be quite useful, if the partner presses the elevated leg against the chest of the person stretching while at the same time holding the opposite leg down on the floor. To do the latter, he may cross his leg over the outstretched leg of the person stretching, at the level of the tibia, in such a way that the leg is held down but not pressured in a way that is uncomfortable.

 The lack of flexibility in the ischiotibial muscles could cause lumbar discomfort, due to the straightening, and even inversion of the natural spinal curvature of the area. Stretching exercises are necessary to prevent this from happening.

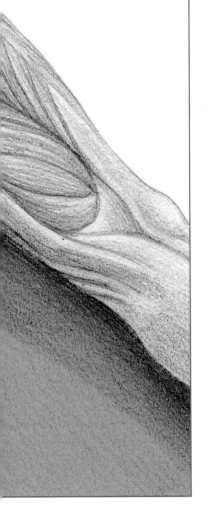

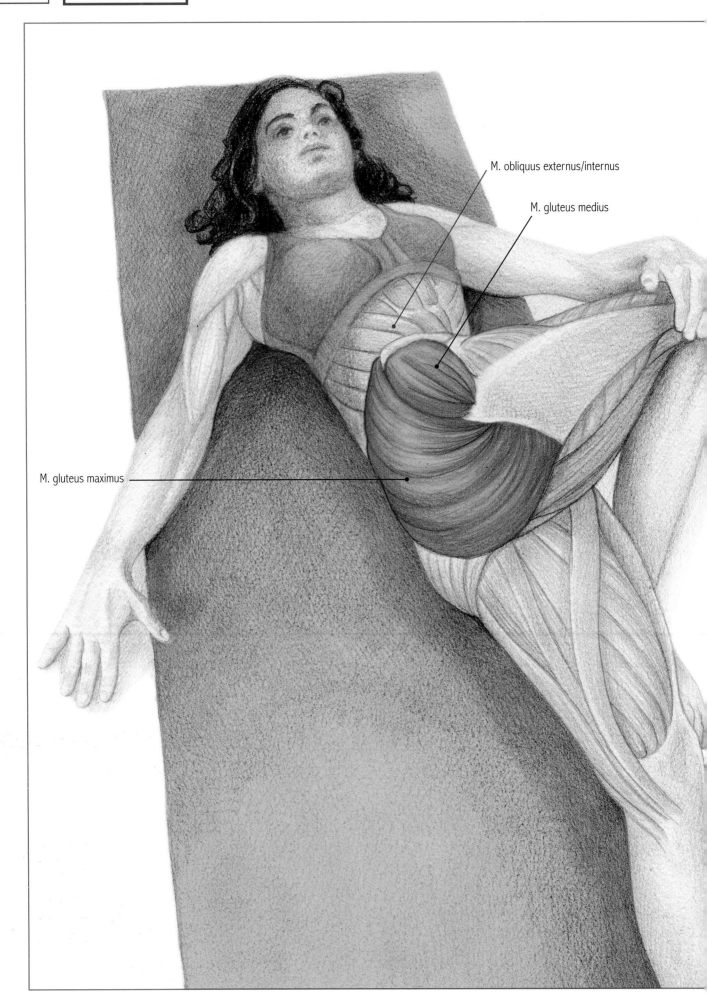

M. obliquus externus/internus

M. gluteus medius

M. gluteus maximus

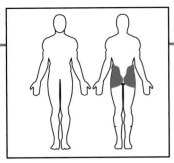

Muscles involved

Principal: Gluteus maximus and medius

Secondary: Abdominal obliques, pyramidal, geminus, obturator externus and obturator internus

Execution

Lying down on the ground, one leg is flexed (both the hip and the knee), and it is taken to the opposite side with the help of the contralateral hand. The opposite arm remains touching the ground completely. The head looks toward the front or even to the side opposite the one where the leg is moving toward, all in an effort to avoid turning the entire trunk.

Comments

People with good flexibility will take the knee right to the ground on the opposite side, always without lifting the non-working arm off the floor or turning the trunk. The stretch is felt in the external area of the gluteus and is very noticeable. It is easy to understand that this exercise involves not only the large muscles that are indicated, but also a whole series of spinal rotator muscles that surround the spine.

If the knee is extended during the execution of this exercise, it will also involve the ischiotibial muscles. If the hip of the elevated leg is flexed even farther it will increase the emphasis upon the pyramidal. One variation to localize the stretch upon the hip (i.e., gluteus medius, tensor fascia lata, etc.) is to place oneself in a position very similar to that of exercise 4.2, but crossing the leg, and not the arm, underneath the body.

This exercise is used, in a similar way, by physiotherapists for the purpose of aligning the spinal column. Therefore, it is likely that some vertebral structures may "crack" when this exercise is performed. This does not seem to pose any particular problem for healthy individuals (see the explanation for exercise 7 in the chapter on forearms and hands).

Variations

13.2... Seated

The position is similar, but now the trunk is straight and the pulling effort upon the knee that moves is greater. This is a very common posture in yoga and is also frequently encountered in sports training.

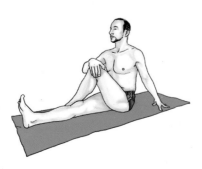

13.3 ...Seated with the leg more extended

The leg that moves remains more extended (both at the hip and at the knee). In this way, there is greater emphasis placed on the gluteus medius and minimus, and not so much on the gluteus maximus.

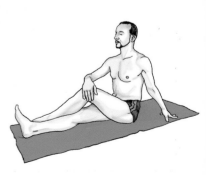

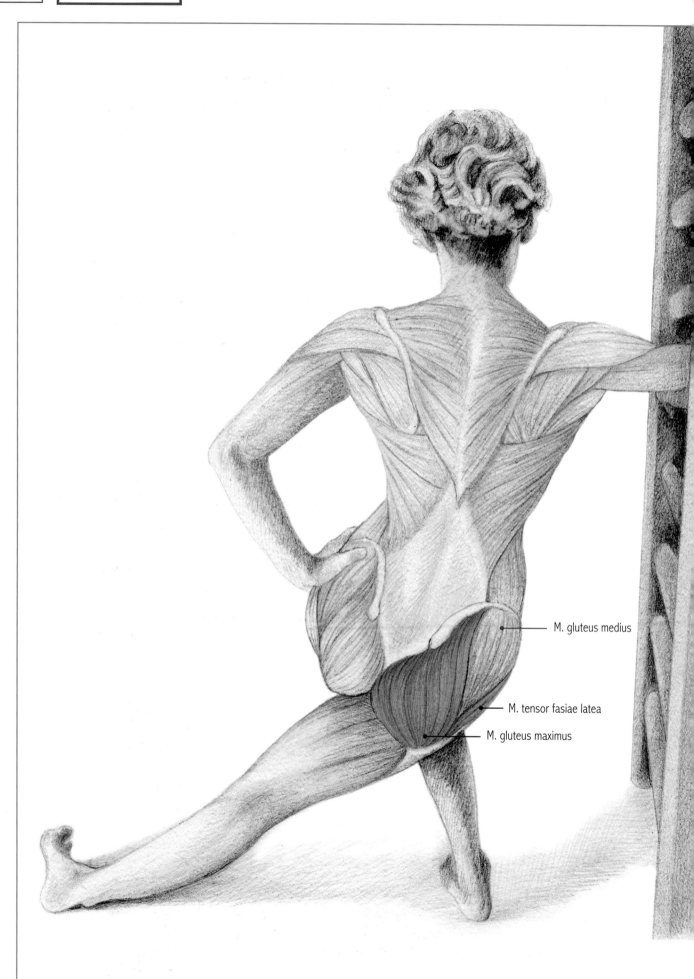

M. gluteus medius

M. tensor fasiae latea

M. gluteus maximus

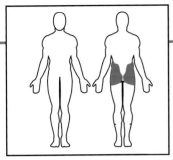

Muscles involved

Principal: Gluteal deltoids (superficial fibers of the gluteus maximus and tensor fascia lata)

Secondary: Gluteus medius

Execution

Standing up, holding on to a support on the side (preferably the wall bars since there are bars at different heights). Release the weight of the body from the leg closest to the support and cross it (in adduction) behind the leg that remains firmly in place. Lower the body slowly at the same time that the free leg is moved into greater adduction.

Comments

Although you will feel significant tension in the area of the gluteus medius in the leg that supports the bodyweight (the great lateral stabilizer of the hip, even in a static standing position), and also of the quadriceps, these are postural tensions rather than true stretches, since the leg that you are really stretching is the other one, the one that was crossed over.

If stretching the adductor muscles is easy, to do the same with the abductor muscles requires positions that are somewhat more uncomfortable, such as the one explained here.

The trunk must remain firm and vertical, never leaning as that would detract from the effectiveness of the exercise. If this exercise is performed correctly, you will notice that the tension runs along the entire lateral area of the leg, from the hip all the way to the knee.

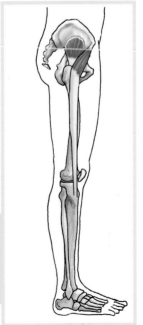

 The principal muscles responsible for the adduction of the hip are the so-called adductors, yet none of the muscles responsible for the abduction of the hip are called "abductors," a common mistake, but rather the "muscles of abduction" or simply by their specific individual names.

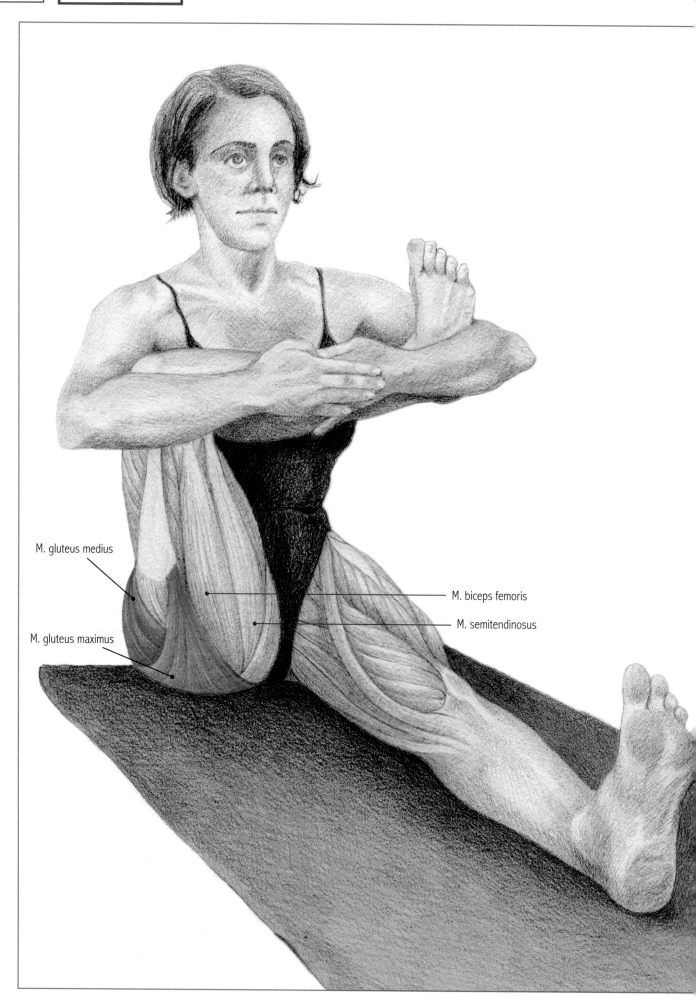

M. gluteus medius

M. gluteus maximus

M. biceps femoris

M. semitendinosus

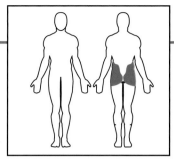

Muscles involved

Principal: Gluteus maximus and medius

Secondary: Pyramidal, ischiotibial muscles

Execution

Seated on the ground, with your back resting against a wall, cross one leg over the other and raise it, bringing it closer to the trunk, like a "hug." The leg on the ground remains extended.

Comments

The arms must cover the entire leg that is being worked, especially the knee, in order to focus the effort on the desired area, which in this case are the gluteus and adjacent muscles. If you only pulled on the feet, the tension upon the knee would be counterproductive.

One variant of this exercise (for some it may be too uncomfortable), consists of the following; stand up in front of a table that is about waist height, flex one leg and support it laterally on top of the table (the lateral zone of the leg), then lean progressively over the table.

The most common mistake consists of flexing the trunk, with the force of the abdominals, in an attempt to diminish the space between the leg and the chest. On the contrary, the back should never come off the wall, and the ischial bones of the hip should be firmly supported on the ground.

 The extended knee cannot rotate, and in flexion it can only do so partially (approximately 30 degrees of internal rotation and roughly 40 degrees of external rotation). The reason is the way in which the ligaments tense when it is extended. Although this is necessary for the stability during walking and running, it is also the main reason behind many of the knee ligament injuries that are seen in certain sports (for example, soccer, skiing, tennis, martial arts, etc.).

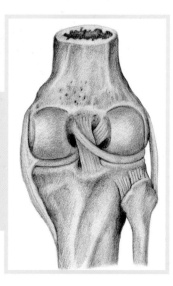

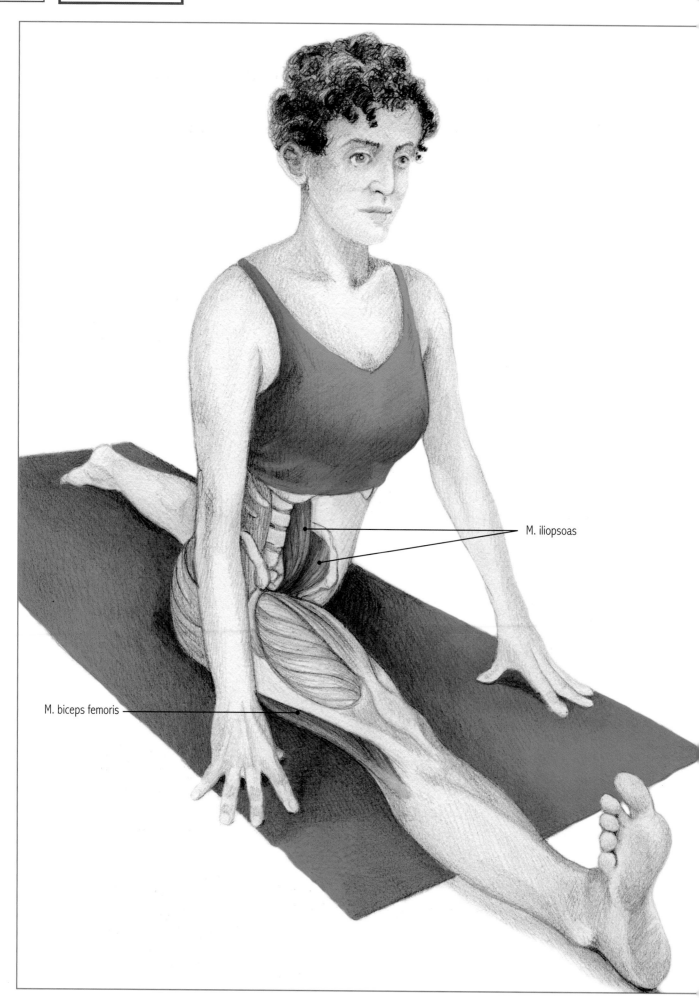

M. iliopsoas

M. biceps femoris

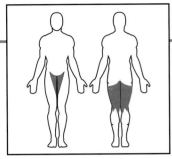

Muscles involved

Principal: Ischiotibial muscles, illiopsoas

Secondary: Adductors, gracilis, sartorius, popliteal, pectineus

Execution

While standing, one leg is brought forward in a very wide stride, and you slowly lower the body closer to the ground while the two legs separate, one in flexion and one in extension. The knees must remain extended and only a slight flexion is permitted in the rear leg. In the final position, the one that must be maintained, the heel of the forward foot is rested on the floor, and the medial surface of the rear foot.

Comments

In this well-known exercise, beginners will not be able to "sit" on the ground, which may create tension on the knees. The measure of how many centimeters are left before touching the ground can serve as an index of improvement throughout the months of training.

The maximum posture is taken to be when the person sits on the ground, but in order to achieve greater degrees of mobility, he may place himself in the air, with the legs on top of two supports (two chairs or two benches, for example). However, this usually proves to the unnecessary because almost no one can reach farther than that in the degree of stretch.

The frontal variant, has been omitted because it forces the knees unnecessarily and does not contribute anything new to the exercise (see exercise 17).

 As a general rule, women are slightly more flexible than men. The reasons for this are many: less bone and muscle mass, preparation for pregnancy and childbirth, hormonal differences, even cultural differences (society has traditionally seen men as having greater strength and women as being more flexible).

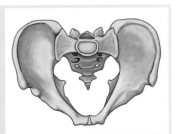

There are exceptions, such as the mandible, where men tend to have greater flexibility, or the fingers of the hand, where they tend to be equal.

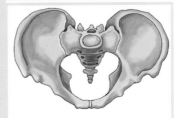

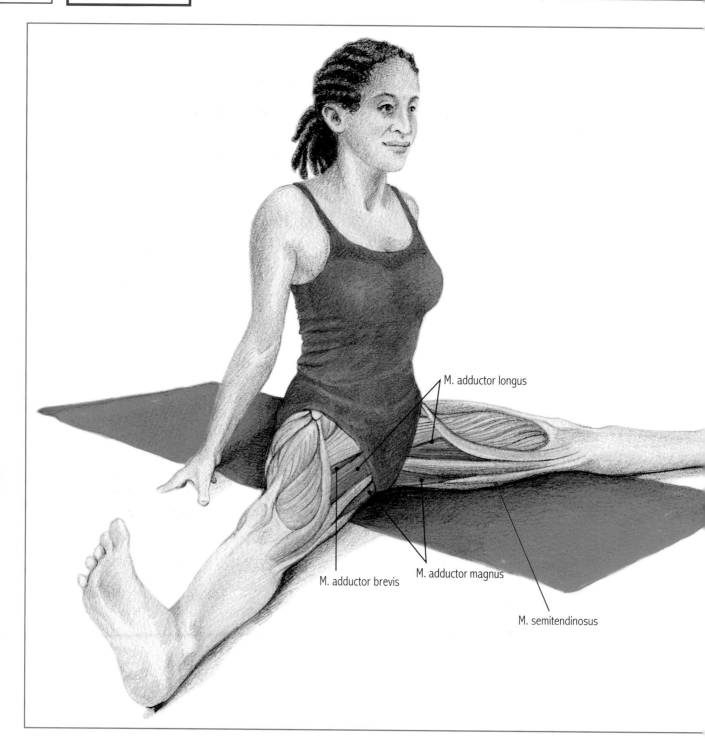

M. adductor longus

M. adductor brevis

M. adductor magnus

M. semitendinosus

Variations | **17.2 ...With flexion to the front**

The posture is basically the same, but upon achieving the desired opening of the legs, the trunk is flexed, bringing it closer to the ground in front of it. The adductors are worked equally, but now there is greater emphasis placed on the extensors of the hip (for example, ischiotibial muscles, gluteus, etc.). One must remember that the turn should be at the hip, rather than at the trunk, hunching the back in order to try to reach farther.

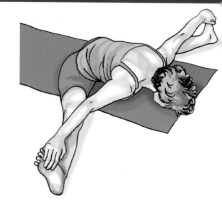

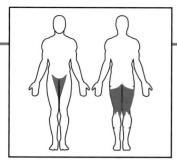

Muscles involved

Principal: Adductor mayor, medius and minor (and minimus when it exists)

Secondary: Gracilis, illiopsoas, ischiotibial muscles

Execution

Seated on the floor, preferably with the back resting on a wall (especially beginners), open the legs in abduction with the knees always extended and the heels resting on the ground.

Comments

This exercise rapidly reveals the flexibility of the adductor muscles. Progressively, with the passage of time, one will have to help with the hands (or a partner) in order to reach an extra centimeter in the opening.

If the ischiotibial muscles hinder the stretching of the adductors, it is enough to simply flex the knees very lightly, separate the gluteus a little bit from the wall in order to extend the hip a little more, or seek variations where these remain flexed (for example, exercise 18). If, on the other hand, we want these muscles to also be stretched, then the knees must be pressed toward the floor (press over the thighs, not direcly over the knees) and keep the trunk straight or slightly flexed.

When this exercise is performed without the support of the wall, the hands must hold the body from behind (as is shown in the image). Since this posture predisposes the hip to extending even farther than if the back is completely supported upon the wall, the resistance offered by the ischiotibial muscles (and the stretch that they receive) tend to be less.

If you are helped by a partner, it is preferable to have him push on the knees to open the legs, rather than pushing on the feet, in order to avoid excessive tension upon one of the ligaments in the area (such as the lateral internal ligament).

17.3 ... With the support of the wall

The posture here is similar to the exercise explained above, but now the back remains against the ground, always with the gluteus against the wall, and the legs extend and open on said wall. This exercise works the same muscles, it is just a matter of which variation a person finds to be more comfortable; and with this last variation, you can achieve a perfect support and alignment of the entire trunk and hip.

The standing variation (frontal split) has been omitted because it does not add anything new to the exercise except putting more pressure upon the knees. Although experienced individuals can perform it without any significant problems.

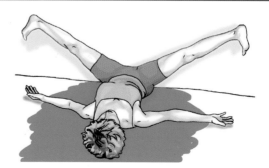

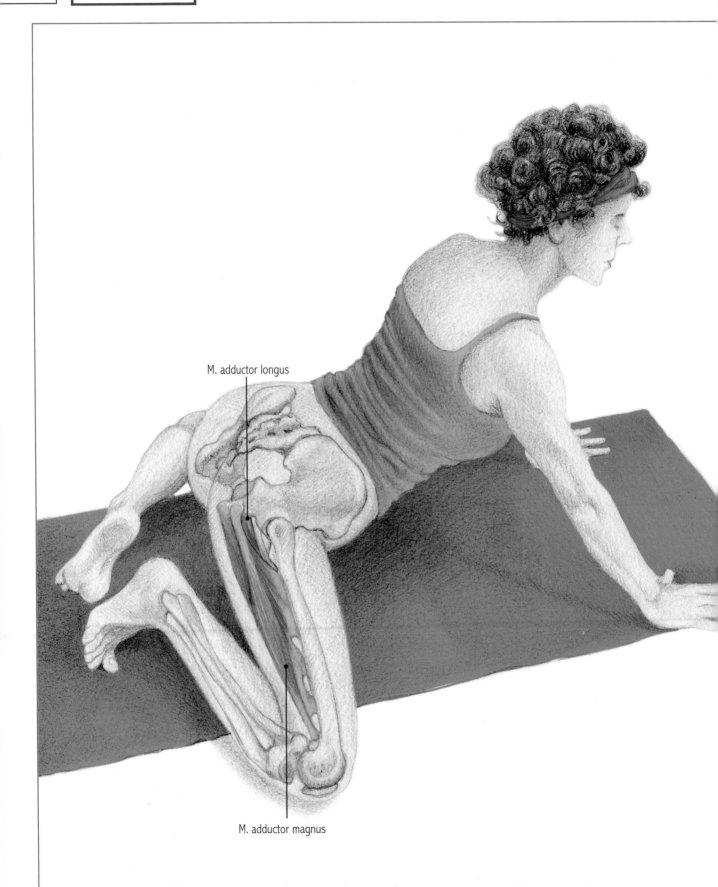

M. adductor longus

M. adductor magnus

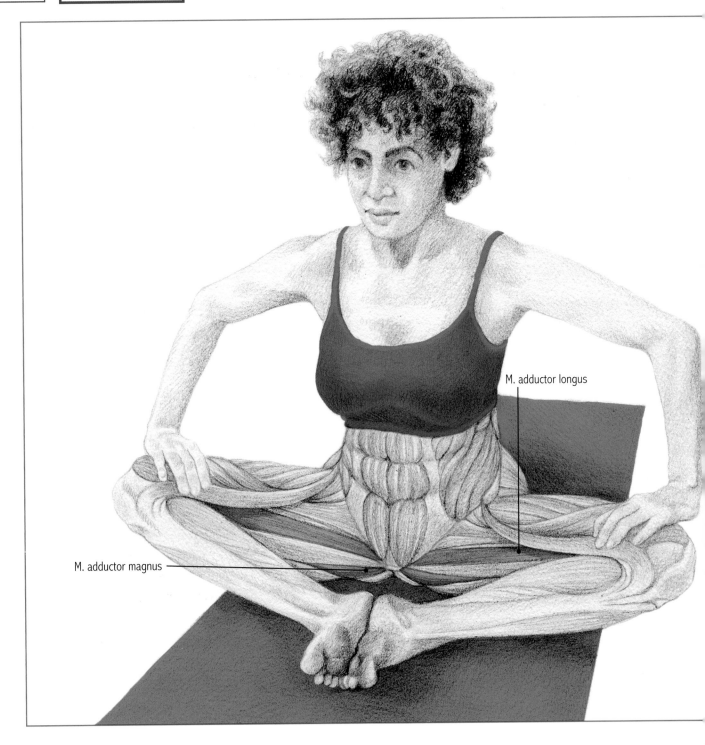

M. adductor longus

M. adductor magnus

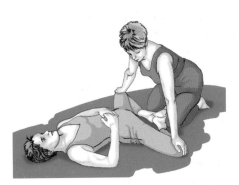

Frequently, the pressure that we exert upon the knees is not enough for the stretching possibilities of this exercise. To seek help, a partner will press on the knees, while the person stretching rests the back on the ground and thereby allows the work of this partner to take effect. The partner will place his knees by the feet to hold them in place, to keep the person who is stretching from extending the legs when he feels the strain.

The position is very good for stretching the set of the adductor muscles (including the gracilis) but the posture must not lead one to elevate the lumbar region off the floor due to the effort. The partner must keep in mind that he has all the strength of his weight to exert upon the knees, and must therefore be careful to gradually increase the pressure so as not to injure the other person.

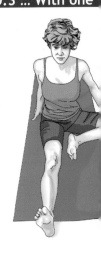

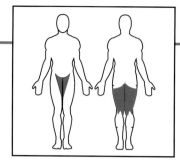

Muscles involved

Principal: Adductors

Secondary: Ischiotibial muscles, gracilis, sartorius, popliteus

Execution

Starting from a standing position, open one leg laterally (abduct it) at the same time that you crouch down upon the other. In the final position, rest over the flexed leg while on the other, rest the heel. One must try to keep the trunk vertical throughout this exercise.

Comments

There are two main muscle groups that are worked in this position: the ischiotibial muscles and the adductors. In order to achieve this, the open leg must remain with the knee extended and sufficiently open. Under no circumstances should you bounce, something that was very commonly done in this exercise a few years ago.

The variation where you do not rest the heel of the foot, but rather the entire medial surface of the foot, is discouraged because of the unnecessary stress it places upon the knee, especially upon the lateral internal ligament. On occasion, the exercise is done standing up, supporting the elevated leg in adduction (internal aspect of the foot over the ground or over a support): the safest way to perform this variation is flexing the knee and resting it over the support, rather than doing it with the knee extended and resting on the foot.

Variation	19.2 ... Over a support

The exercise is similar, except that now you remain standing up and rest the leg on an elevated support (better if it is padded). Here, the posture makes one more prone to rest the internal aspect of the foot; something that should be avoided in general, just like it was explained in the main exercise.

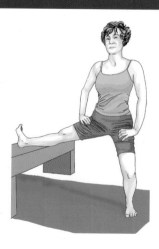

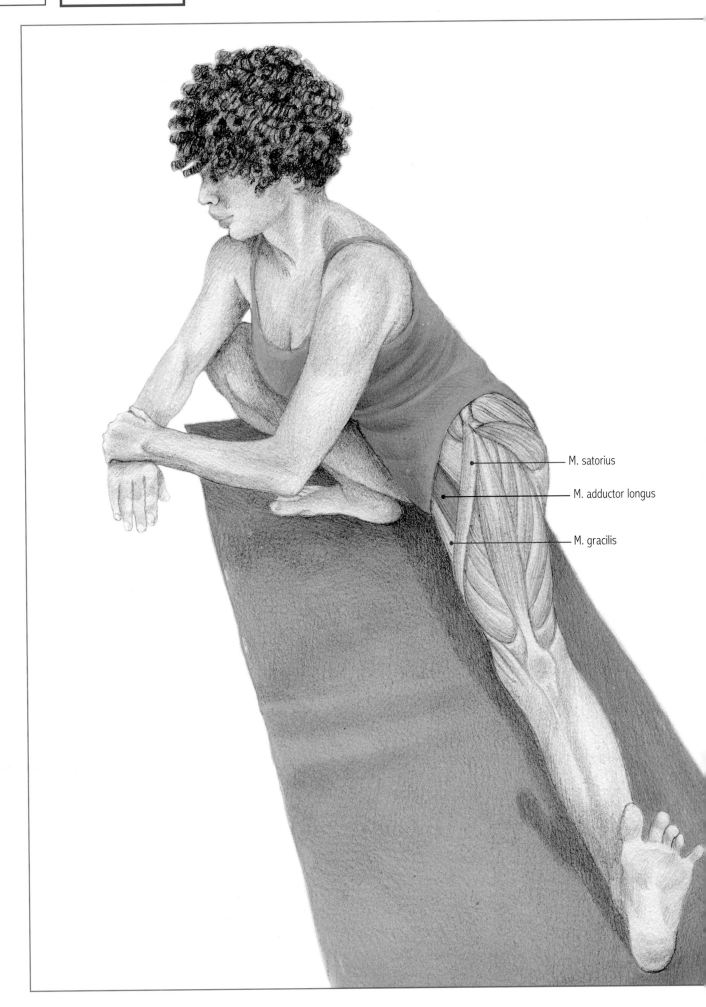

M. satorius

M. adductor longus

M. gracilis

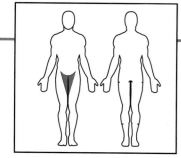

Muscles involved

Principal: Adductor major and medius

Secondary: Adductor minor (illiopsoas)

Execution

Place yourself on the ground on a padded mat resting the hands and knees on the floor, and open the hip by separating the knees from each other in such a way that the pelvis gets closer to the floor. When you reach the lowest point, you can rest the forearms and elbows on the ground, instead of the hands, in order to achieve a more comfortable posture and avoid having the back curve in hyperlordosis.

Comments

The pelvis is lowered vertically; one must not make the mistake of lowering it toward the back as if you were going to sit on your heels, which would take away from the stretching of the adductors. Only when the bony parts of the hip meet one another, can you then vary the flexion slightly in order to continue with the movement.

Given that the very weight of the hip is not enough to produce a sufficient stretch, we will have to make use of our own muscular strength in order to "push" it downward. A partner could help by applying a light pressure over the hip, but being careful not to rest all of his bodyweight upon it.

We must refrain from performing this exercise on anything but a padded surface, otherwise the hips will suffer too much. Furthermore, it should be pointed out that in a sharp or forced abduction, the rectus femoris is the adductor most likely to be injured.

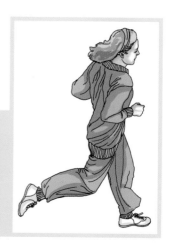

 The phenomenon known as cellulitis does not improve with stretching exercises. All the indications point to the fact that it will not disappear even if we stretch it, press it, massage it, heat it or cool it. In addition to surgery, only diet and aerobic exercise can significantly improve the abnormal accumulation of fat and liquids in certain body areas.

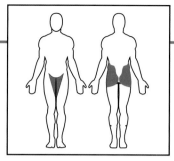

Muscles involved

Principal: Gluteus maximus and medius

Secondary: Adductors

Execution

Starting from a standing position, crouch down without lifting the bottoms of the feet off the ground until the hip gets close to the ground.

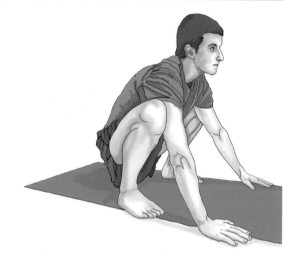

Comments

To keep your balance, the body should remain in between the legs and the arms should remain forward, although people with good mobility at the hip and the ankles can place themselves without any problems with the arms on the outside of the legs. Once you have found your equilibrium point, it is advisable to relax and maintain that posture. Bouncing is not recommended.

A small variation consists of placing the feet facing outward at a 45° angle and pressing with the elbows outward on the knees, to put more emphasis on the adductors.

If you find it difficult to maintain your balance, it is also useful to hold on to something stable in front of you (for example, wall bars or something similar), and let the weight of the body fall backwards and down.

People who suffer from knee pains should avoid this exercise, since the flexion of the knees supporting weight over 90° can be counterproductive.

 This position is often adopted by children and adults in order to rest while crouching down. However, a bad posture or, especially lifting weight from this position, could stress certain ligaments, like the ones in the knee, or the meniscus of the knee.

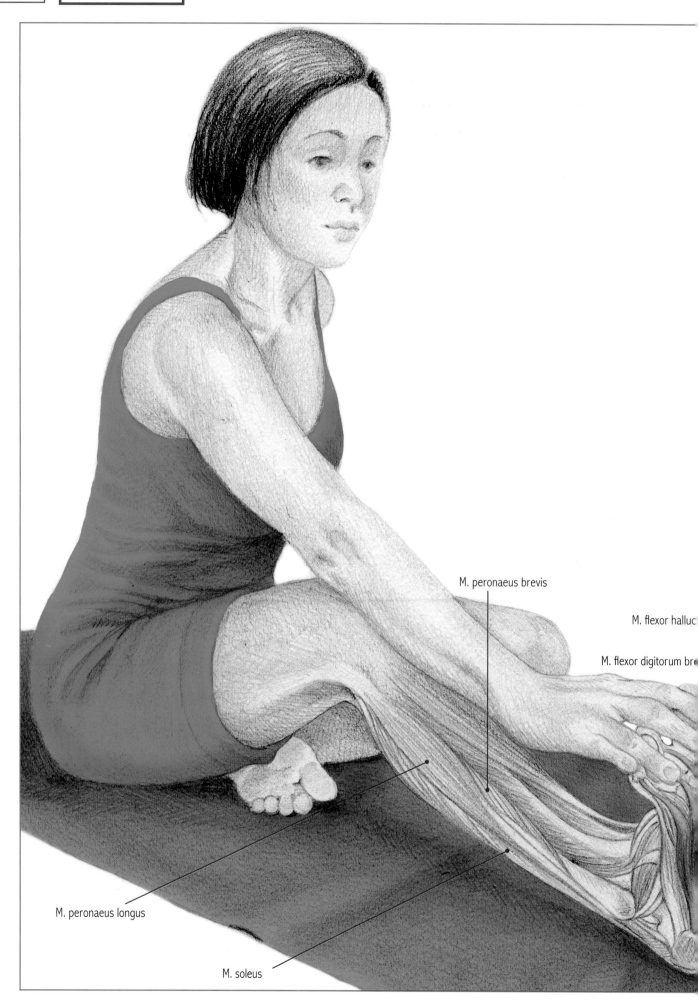

M. peronaeus brevis

M. flexor halluc

M. flexor digitorum br

M. peronaeus longus

M. soleus

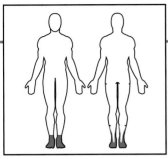

Muscles involved

Principal: Flexor digitorum longus and flexor digitorum brevis

Secondary: Soleus, plantaris, peroneus (gastrocnemius)

Execution

Seated on the ground or on a bench, flex the foot toward the tibia with the help of the hand. In principle, the hand covers a great part of the sole of the foot in order to produce a general flexion, but varying the zone that is flexed, we will work one area or another in the manner that is explained below.

Comments

If the flexion is performed with the knee extended, then the stretch will focus especially on the gastrocnemius and soleus, whereas if the knee is flexed, it will focus on the latter.

On the other hand, if the traction is solely upon the toes, the intensity of the stretch will be greatest upon the flexor digitorum longus and brevis, as well as the lumbricals. All these different variations should be performed to ensure that they are all properly stretched.

This exercise, when it is performed with the knee extended, substitutes the exercise performed while standing on a step or on the ground (exercises 25 and 26). The advantage here is that when applying pressure with the hand, it is gentler and more controlled than simply releasing all of your bodyweight upon the heel of the foot. The disadvantage is that not everyone posseses the flexibility that is required to perform this exercise, the ischiotibial muscles could prevent the person from being able to hold on to his feet with the knee extended, and must, therefore, return to the above-mentioned exercises.

 The Compartment Syndrome due to overload is common among sprinters, especially when it is done over inadequate surfaces. The tibial muscle, possibly already hypertrophied, becomes inflamed and compresses the blood vessels and nerves. The stretches and massages of the tibial region can, in many cases, prevent and sometimes improve this injury. The prevention, with an unhurried racing technique, frequent rests, adequate footwear and a proper surface on which to run, are the best advice.

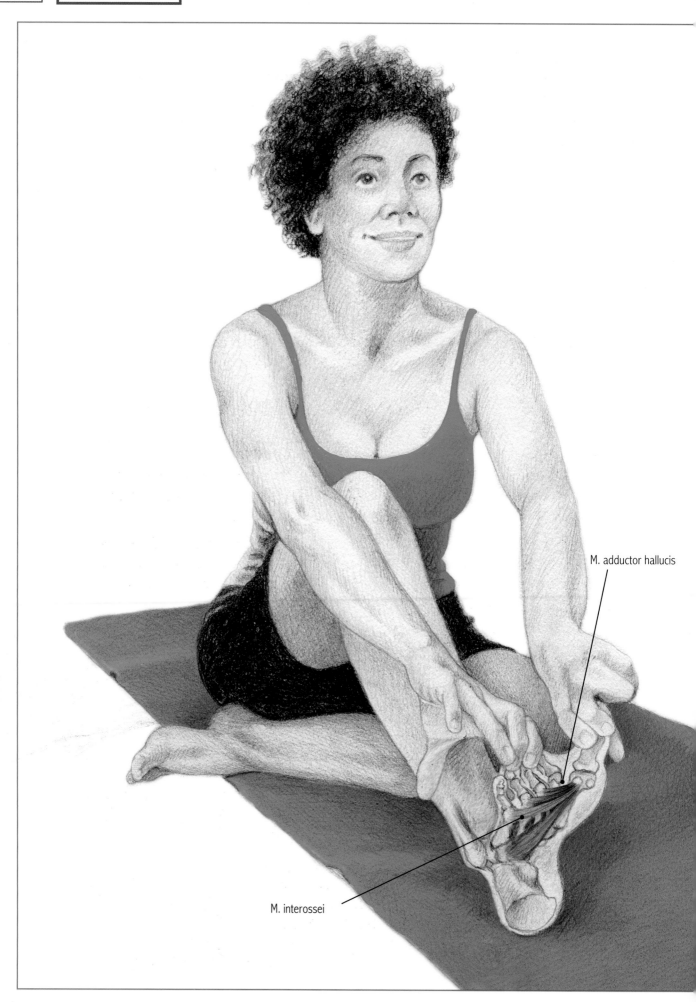

M. adductor hallucis

M. interossei

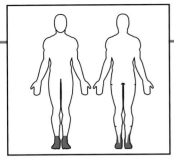

Muscles involved

Principal: Plantar interosseus, adductor hallucis

Secondary: Various ligaments of the foot

Execution

This uncommon and fairly complicated exercise consists of separating each pair of toes one by one, with the help of the hands.

Comments

Although this may not be a basic exercise, since it doesn't stretch muscles or structures that need stretching on a frequent basis, it is true that on occasion, the footwear will press upon, or at least immobilize the toes, and so it is important to regain this lost mobiity with exercises such as this one.

Walking around barefoot, especially on the sand at the beach, can be a pleasant and valid alternative, although not as specific or as strict as moving each toe individually. In any case, footwear should never harm the toes, ankle or any other part of the body, because let's remember that a poor support has repercussions in many other areas of the body (the knees, the hips, the spine, etc.).

 In contrast with other primates, human beings have toes that are very atrophied. There is a theory that says the 5th toes are even disappearing in our species. But for the moment, it is known that they play an important role in the static and dynamic stability of the body, and so we must try to keep them strong, healthy and flexible.

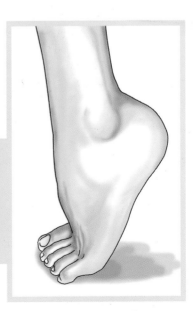

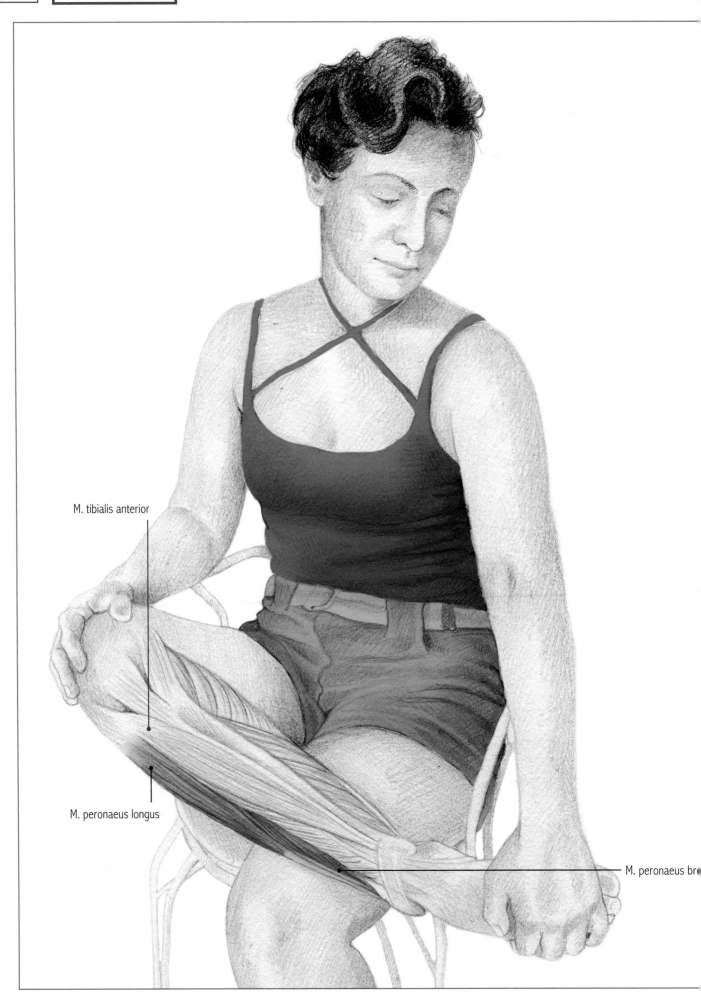

M. tibialis anterior

M. peronaeus longus

M. peronaeus br

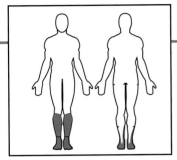

Muscles involved

Principal: Peroneus

Secondary: Tibialis anterior and tibialis posterior

Execution

Seated on the ground or on a bench, move the foot in such a way as to cause the stretching of its different areas. The position of flexion and extension of the ankle are explained earlier in the book (see exercises 5 to 9).

Comments

Each stretching position must be held for a few seconds, and so we must not just simply turn the foot in all different directions (circumduction), but rather adopt a position of tension and hold it for a time and then change to a different one. The muscles and tendons that are mobilized are very varied and beyond the scope of this book, here we have only pointed out the basics.

The ankle is one of the most fragile joints, along with the knee, when it comes to practicing sports. Its strenghtening, stretching, and proprioception (self-perception of its position and movement) are essential for a healthy joint and for preventing problems in the future. In this exercise, it is necessary to know how to relax the different muscles that surround the ankle, since any tension will take away from the effectiveness of the stretching exercise.

 In the leg and foot, we find muscles and ligaments that are incredibly strong, and the reason is obvious. They are supporting the weight of the entire body structure. Just like the pillars in a building are thicker and more resistent in the lower floors than in the upper floors, human beings are designed to be able to vertically support all their weight, and when it reaches the foot, to spread the load over its surface. Therein lies the importance of a good stride and of maintaining the muscles and ligaments in good equilibrium between strength and flexibility.

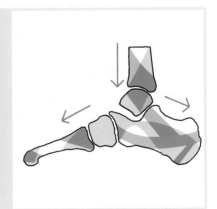

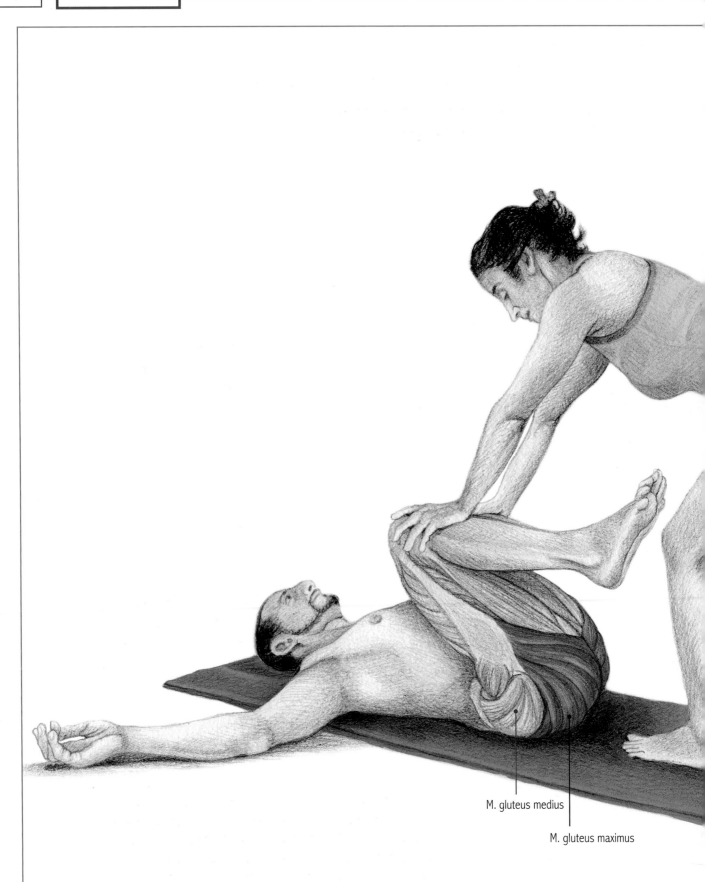

M. gluteus medius

M. gluteus maximus

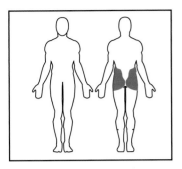

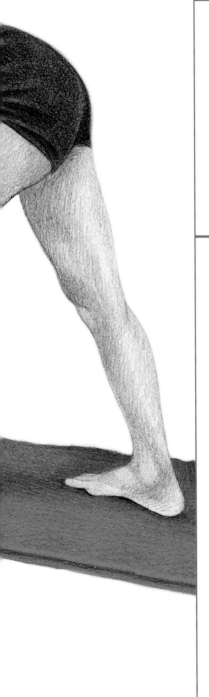

Muscles involved

Principal: Gluteus maximus

Secondary: Gluteus medius

Execution

The person stretching lies down comfortably on the floor in a decubitus supine position (on his back), preferably over a pad, brings the legs together and flexes the hip and the knees. The training partner presses the knees against his partner's chest, applying the pushing force over the tibial region.

Comments

The training partner must not hold back when it comes to unloading a great portion of his bodyweight upon the legs of the person performing the stretch since this is an exercise with a low risk of injury and/or or feeling pain. The only precaution will be to keep in mind that the pelvis should not lift off the floor in order to maintain good stability in the spinal column.

Although this exercise produces a deep flexion of the hip, the ischiotibial muscles are barely stretched, since the knees remain bent.

* In spite of what one may read in some sporting articles or books, neither the strongest muscles nor the best planned stretches can avoid an injury to the meniscus or ligaments of the knee if it suffers a strong rotation in extension, as may occur in some sports where when you run, you plant the foot and turn the waist. From the point of view of the bones, the stability of the knee is scarce. In case of an injury, the immediate treatment involves rest, elevation, ice and compression.

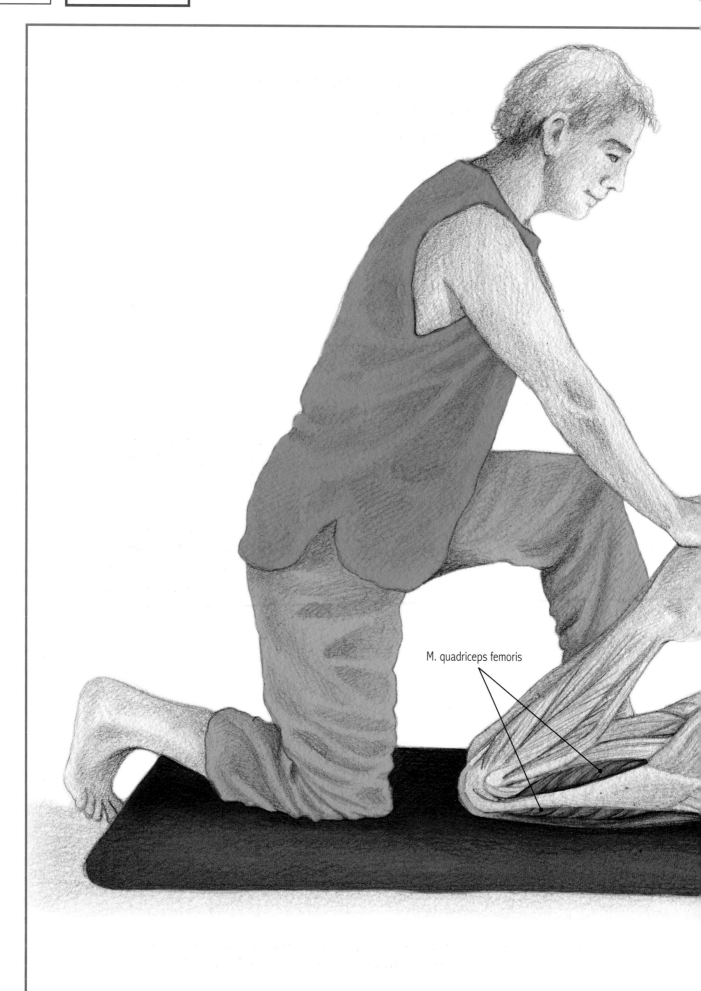

M. quadriceps femoris

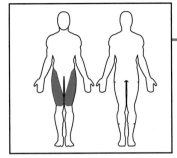

Muscles involved

Principal: Quadriceps
Secondary: Illiopsoas

Execution

The person performing the stretch lies down in a decubitus prone position (face down) and flexes the knees. The training partner presses upon the metatarsals of the feet of his partner in such a way that he brings them closer to the gluteus.

Comments

As was the case with the previous exercise, here the risk of injury is almost nonexistent, what's more, the majority of people will notice that they are able to touch their gluteus with the heel of the foot. The partner should, therefore, unload almost all of his bodyweight upon the person performing the stretch, who at no point should feel any pain.

Of the four vastus muscles of the quadriceps, the rectus femoris is the one that is stressed the least during this stretch, since the position of the hip is aligned with the knee, not extended. There is a small variation other one free, for now), flex the knee completely with one hand while with the other hand he holds it from underneath. From that position — and without extending the joint — elevate the knee from the ground lightly. This variation should not be performed with both legs at the same time, or you will inevitably turn the hip, nullifying the stretch you try to achieve.

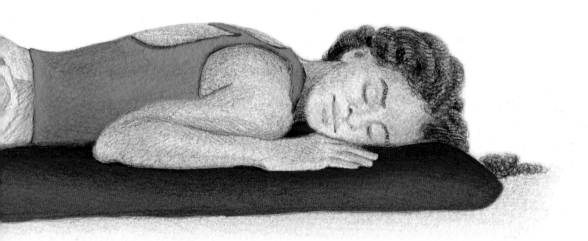

 In many sporting activities the competition is healthy and even necessary. But when it comes to stretching, competition to see who can achieve the greater gains is not a good idea as it could lead to injury.

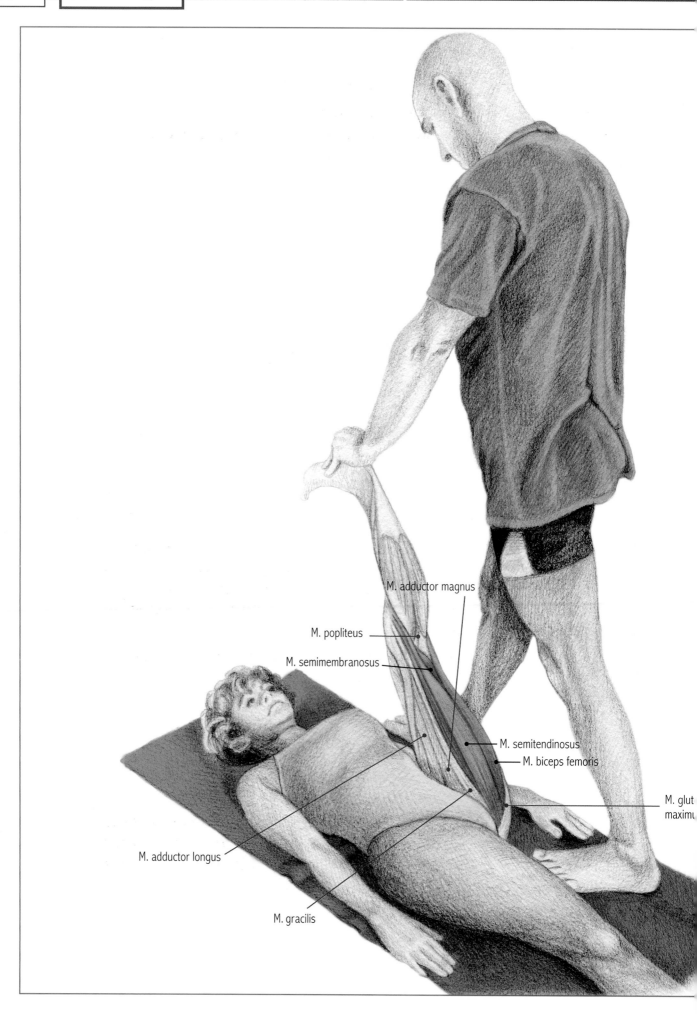

M. adductor magnus

M. popliteus

M. semimembranosus

M. semitendinosus

M. biceps femoris

M. glut
maximu

M. adductor longus

M. gracilis

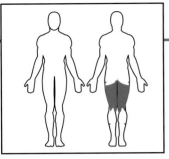

Muscles involved

Principal: Ischiotibial muscles

Secondary: Gluteus maximus, sartorius, popliteus, gracilis, adductors, illiopsoas

Execution

The person performing the stretch lies down on the floor, preferably over a padded mat. The partner takes one of the legs and, always with the knee extended, raises it in flexion of the hip.

Comments

People with little flexibility will have difficulty keeping the other leg on the ground, and they will rapidly notice how their illiopsoas muscle also pulls to flex the hip. The training partner must watch out so that this does not occur, placing one of his feet on top of the outstretched leg if necessary. Another point to keep in mind as the training partner is that the leg that is being stretched must keep the knee extended, but one doesn`t have to press directly upon it to achieve this, but rather over the thigh.

Only advanced practitioners will be able to hold this position without help, whereas the rest will need help in order to make progress.

 The appropriate intensity in a stretching exercise is when the intense pulling sensation upon reaching the theoretical maximum point gives way after 4 or 5 seconds and becomes more bearable. If the exercise is performed roughly, you will never reach that point. The communication between the training partners is essential to achieve an effective intensity in the stretches.

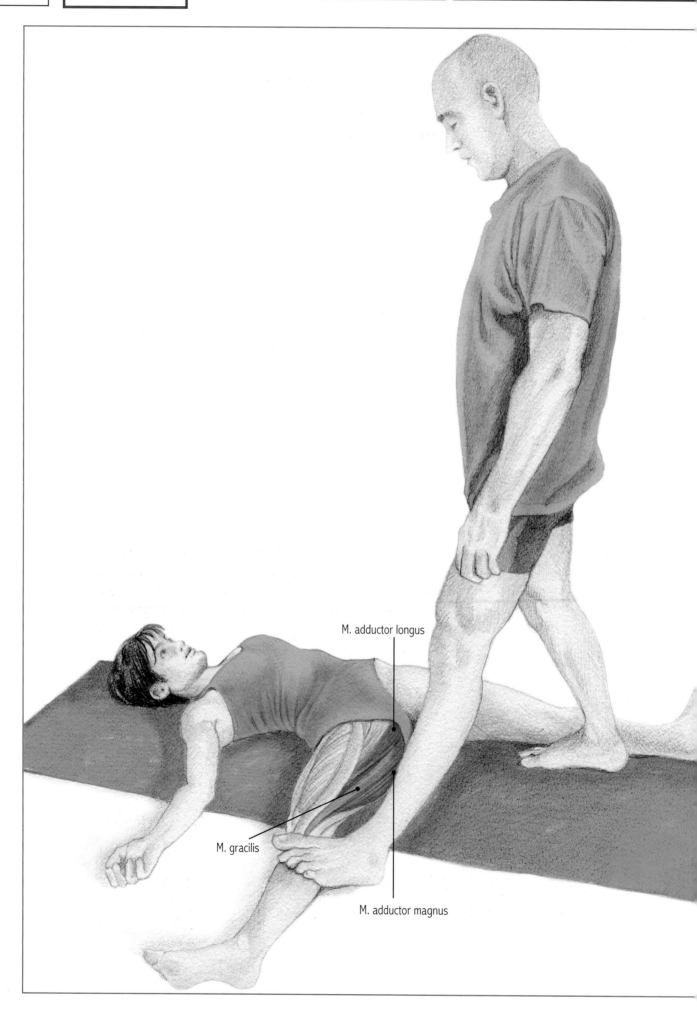

M. adductor longus

M. gracilis

M. adductor magnus

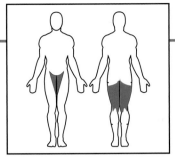

Muscles involved

Principal: Adductors, gracilis

Secondary: Ischiotibial muscles

Execution

Lying on the ground, preferably on a padded mat, the training partner places himself between the two legs of his partner at the level of his knees. He places one of his feet firmly on the ground to immobilize one of the legs of the person executing the stretch, and with the other he opens the leg in abduction.

Comments

The push upon the leg that is being worked (the one that opens up) can be equally done with the hands. The results are better if the partner tries to always keep the knees extended so that both the adductors and the knee flexors will be stretched (biceps femoris, semimembranosus, semitendinosus). The pressure to open the leg should be applied at the knee, rather than the foot, in order to avoid unnecessary tensions over some of the knee ligaments (especially the lateral internal ligament). Let's also remember that the injury to the lateral internal ligaments occurs more commonly than injuries to the external ones, even though they are thicker, because during either walking or running, the knee tends to open up to the inside due to the bony shape.

 In soccer, just to mention a sport that is played commonly, the common belief is that the quadriceps is the most important muscle, but there are two more that deserve special mention: the illiopsoas and the adductors. Any training that ignores these muscles will end up resulting in discomfort or injuries in different areas, from the lumbar region to the pubic bone.

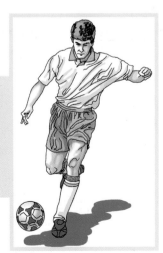

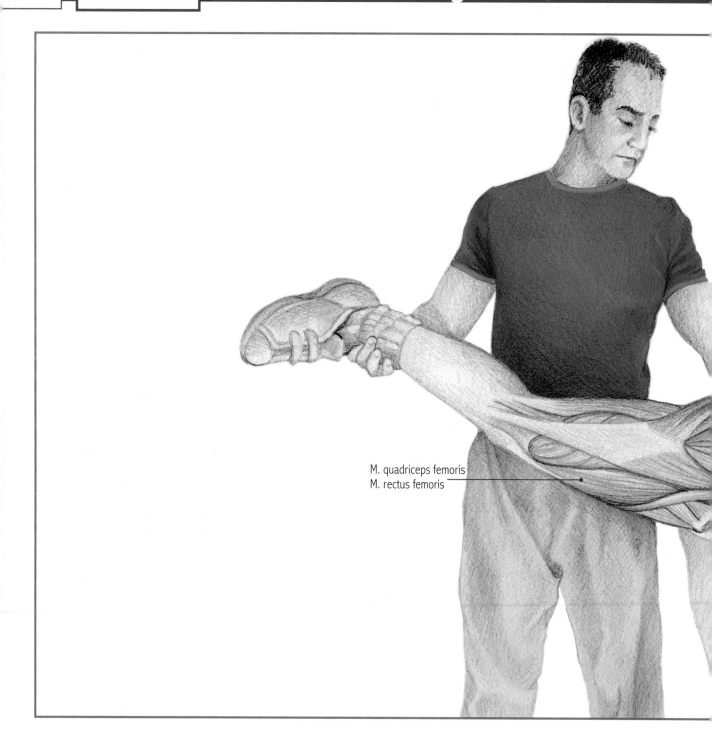

M. quadriceps femoris
M. rectus femoris

Comments

Due to the weight of the leg and the tension of the muscles being worked, the training partner must ha
the strength necessary in order to help perform the exercise, because otherwise it would be a bet
alternative to select a different exercise (for example, see exercise 6). If in addition to the weight of the l
the person performing the stretch does not manage to relax all of the flexor muscles of the hip (especia
the illiopsoas and the rectus femoris), the difficulty for applying a correct level of tension, on the part
the training partner, will be even better.

There is one less useful variation, which is likewise performed in the same manner, but directly on t
floor. The problem is that the hyperlordosis that will be produced when the leg is elevated, so it is r
recommended to pull on both legs at the same time.

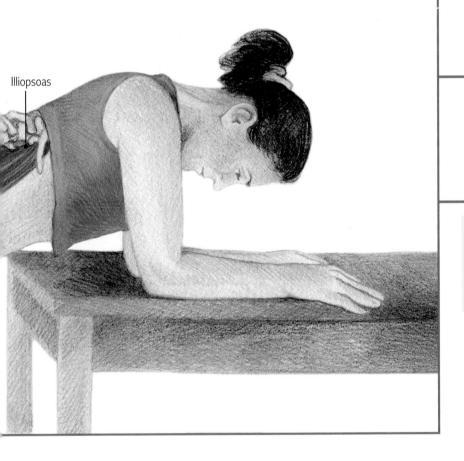

Illiopsoas

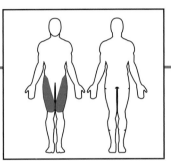

Muscles involved

Principal: Illiopsoas
Secondary: Rectus femoris

Execution

Lying with the stomach over a bench or some other padded support (in a decubitus prone postion), so that the hip remains at the border of same, the partner raises one of the legs in extension.

 It seems like a proven fact that the lack of flexibility of the ischiotibial muscles is one of the causative factors of low back pain in adults. Furthermore, due to the lack of mobility of the hip during our day-to-day lives, these muscles are one of the ones that most quickly suffer contractures and stiffness as the years go by.

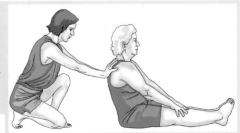

7

Abdomen & Lower Back Group

Descriptive anatomy of the abdomen: biomechanical introduction to the principal muscles

superficial view

deep view

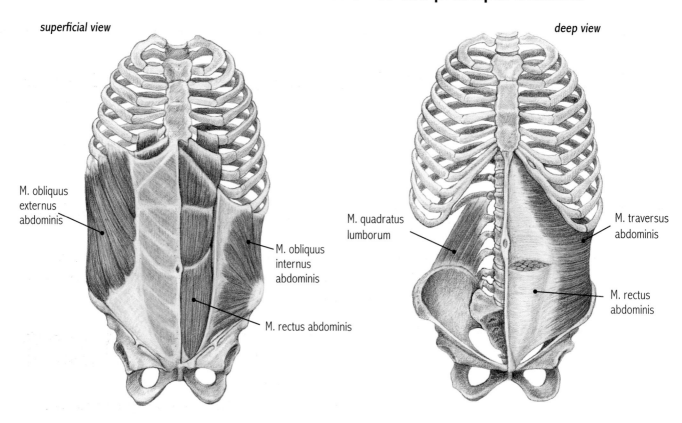

M. obliquus externus abdominis

M. obliquus internus abdominis

M. rectus abdominis

M. quadratus lumborum

M. traversus abdominis

M. rectus abdominis

Flexors

Rectus abdominis (anterior, superficial)

Origin: Ribs 5, 6, and 7; xyphoid process of the sternum

Insertion: Pubic bone (symphisis pubis and lateral expansions)

Principal functions: Flexion of the trunk toward the front, bringing torso and pelvis closer together

External oblique (anterior, superficial)

Origin: Ribs (last 7 or 8 ribs)

Insertion: Illiac crest, crural arch

Principal functions: Flexion of the trunk; lateral leaning to ipsilateral side and rotation of the contralateral side (if it acts on just one side); lowers the ribs

Transversus abdominis (antero-lateral, deep)

Origin: Lumbar vertebrae (vertices of the spinous processes)

Insertion: Pubic bone (superior border of the symphysis pubis and pubis)

Principal functions: Constrains the natural abdominal girdle

Internal oblique (anterior, medium)

Origin: Ribs (last 4)

Insertion: Crural arch, illiac crest, lumbar aponeurosis

Principal functions: Flexion of the trunk, lateral inclination and rotation of its side (if it acts unilaterally); Lowering the ribs

Illiopsoas (anterior, deep)

See "LEGS"

Brief comments: The abdominal muscles play an important role in a countless number of actions, since they move the trunk or fixate it so that it can serve as a support for other movements. Unlike other muscles, these do not need to be stretched as frequently, nor taken to their limits, normally they remain hypotonic at rest.

Descriptive anatomy of the muscles of the lower back: biomechanical introduction to the principal muscles.

Extensors

cro-lumbar (posterior, deep)

gin: Cervical vertebrae (transverse processes of the last 5)

ertion: Sacrum and illiac crests, expansions towards the last 10

ncipal functions: Extension of the trunk; lateral flexion if it acts aterally

rvical, thoracic and lumbar illiocostals (posterior, deep)

gin; Ribs (at the angles of the 3rd to 6th, the cervical); 6 last ribs their angles; the thoracic); sacrum, illeum and T11 and T12 plus bar vertebrae (at the spinous processes; the lumbar)

ertion: Cervical vertebrae (transverse processes C4 – C6, the vical); cervical vertebrae (transverse process of C7) and ribs gles of the first 6, the dorsal); last ribs (angles of the last 6 or 7; lumbar)

ncipal functions: Extension of the vertebral column; flexion and ation to its side if they act unilaterally

uadratus lumborum (posterior, deep)

gin: Illeum (crest, on the posterior-medial one-third of the internal um)

ncipal functions: Lateral flexion of the trunk; collaborates in the ion and extension of the trunk, raises the pelvis laterally.

Longissimus thoracis (posterior, deep)

Origin: Thoracic and lumbar vertebrae (transverse processes)

Insertion: Sacrum and illiac crests

Principal functions: Extension of the vertebral column, lateral flexion and rotation of its side if it acts unilaterally

Trasnversus spinosum (posterior, deep)

Origin: Vertebral lamina

Insertion: Vertebrae (transverse processes of the 4 subjacent vertebrae)

Principal functions: Extension, lateral inclination, rotation of the trunk, active ligament

Serratus minor posterior and inferior (posterior-inferior, deep)

Origin: Ribs (external inferior border of the last 3 or 4 ribs)

Insertion: Thoracic and lumbar vertebrae (spinous processes of the first 3)

Principal functions: Extension, lateral inclination and rotation of the trunk

Latissimus dorsi (posterior, superficial)

(see "Back")

Brief comments: As most people know, the posterior muscles of the spinal column are the "posture" muscles. Everyone knows that the type of lifestyle, at times due to excess work, and others by default, tend to be targets for pains and tensions: The causes of the pains in the lower back can be summarized by the following:

1. Sustained posture: almost always for spending too much time either sitting or standing up.

2. Weakness in the area: due to lack of exercise and muscle tone.

3. Rigidity: due to lack of stretching and mobility.

4. Poor education concerning mobiltity (for example, inappropriate weight increases).

Once the main causes have been identified, it is easy to deduce the principal solutions: education about posture, movement and the practice of physical exercise. It seems paradoxical that, although it is one of the most important muscle groups in the human body, it is so frequently ignored and forgotten.

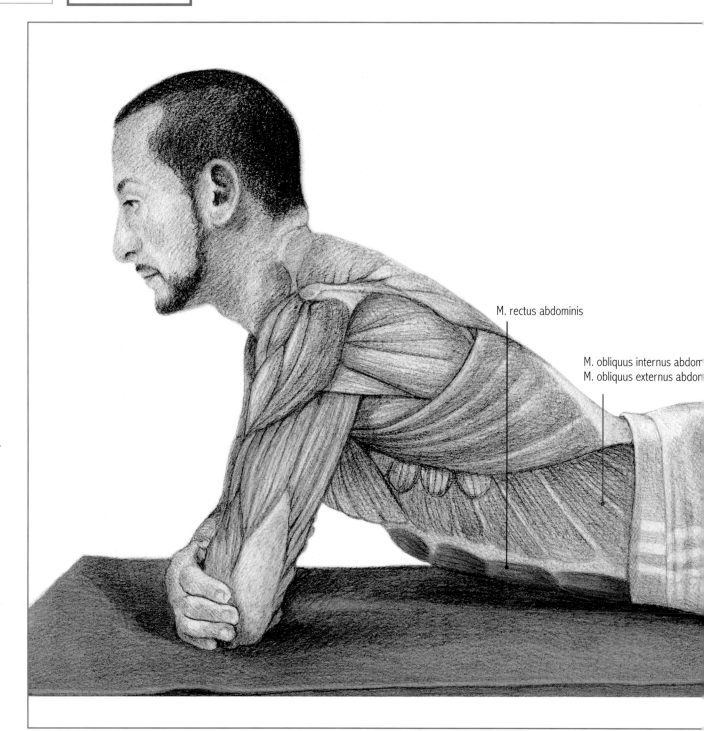

M. rectus abdominis

M. obliquus internus abdom
M. obliquus externus abdor

Variation **1.2... Over the hands**

This variation tends to be the most commonly practiced, and even the most commonly explained in some manuals. However, in addition to an unmecessary degree of stretching to which the rectus abdominus is subjected, the vertebral processes (especially in the lumbar region) may crash inappropriately. Not all the spinous processes are of the same length, they are shorter in the lumbar region than in the thoracic region for example, which is one of the reasons you are able to extend the lumbar more than the thoracic region. But not everyone has the same length spinous processes, nor is the space between them the same for all individuals. Therefore, some people may be much more comfortable extending their spinal column than others, and do so with less risk.

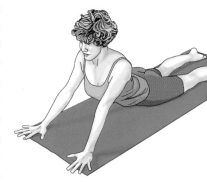

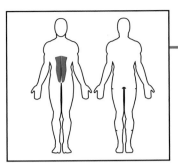

Muscles involved

Principal: Rectus abdominus

Secondary: Abdominal obliques, transverse abdominus

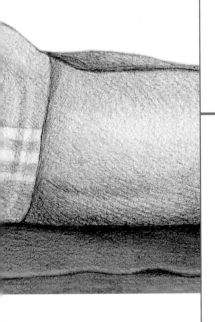

Execution

Lying face down on the floor (decubitus prone position), elevate the trunk and support yourself over the elbows in such a way that you feel a gentle tension over the abdomen.

Comments

As it is known, the rectus abdominus is a muscle that does not need a lot of stretching; it is enough with exercises like the one pictured here in order to exercise it normally. This does not mean that it should not be stretched periodically, since the excessive tension in many sporting activities, even the specific training to which it is normally subjected, may cause some pain in different areas, such as the lower back for example.

ıt there are motives other than uneasiness, such as the unnecessary stress to ıich the intervertebral discs are subjected; thick and sufficiently strong in the ınbar region to be able to support all of the bodyweight, but to which a yawning the vertebrae implies an unbalanced stress.

:hough each person tends to know his or her limits, in this exercise it is not commended that you try to improve this posture.

rtainly there is no problem in performing it ocassionally, but the professional vice of the author is to avoid it for the reasons explained above.

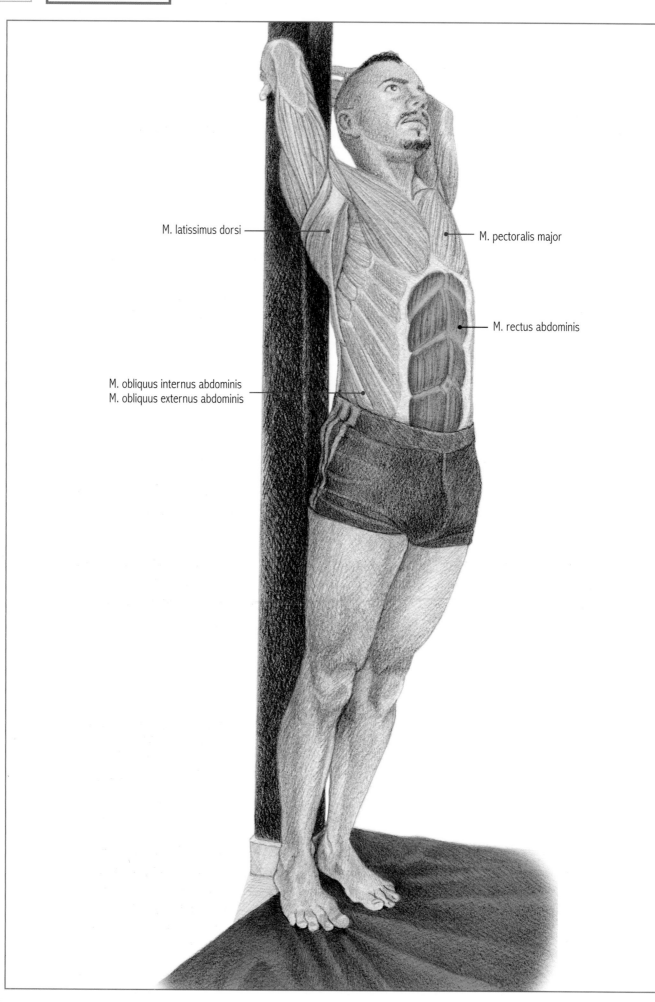

M. latissimus dorsi

M. pectoralis major

M. rectus abdominis

M. obliquus internus abdominis
M. obliquus externus abdominis

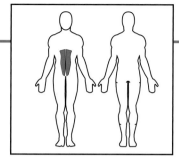

Muscles involved

Principal: Rectus abdominus

Secondary: Abdominal obliques, transverse abdominus, latissimus dorsi, pectoralis major, teres major

Execution

Place yourself with your back to a column or another similar support (wall bars are also good), with the whole body against the support. Hold on with your hands over your head and let the body fall forward gently, without moving the feet.

Comments

This exercise provides enough of a stretch over the abdominal group, but also over other important muscles such as the latissimus dorsi and the triceps. The position of the body must be relaxed, there is no need to make any effort in an attempt to take the exercise further.

The variation where one holds on to a horizontal bar, over the head and not from the back, is also valid. In this case, it must be high enough so that the body can touch the ground without any difficulty, and from there let yourself fall forward without moving the feet from their original position. The final position is very similar to the exercise here explained, the only difference being that the arms are over the head.

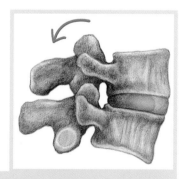

 During many movements of the spinal column, a partial "pinching" of the intervertebral discs is produced, especially during movements of flexion and extension. In healthy individuals and young people, the tolerance levels are greater, but with increasing age, both inadequate postures and movements are no longer well absorbed by the discs, and this is the reason why some (above all the lumbar hyperextension) must be avoided. The meeting of the spinous processes is a second reason why all these exercises that involve a lot of extension must be performed with extreme caution or not performed at all.

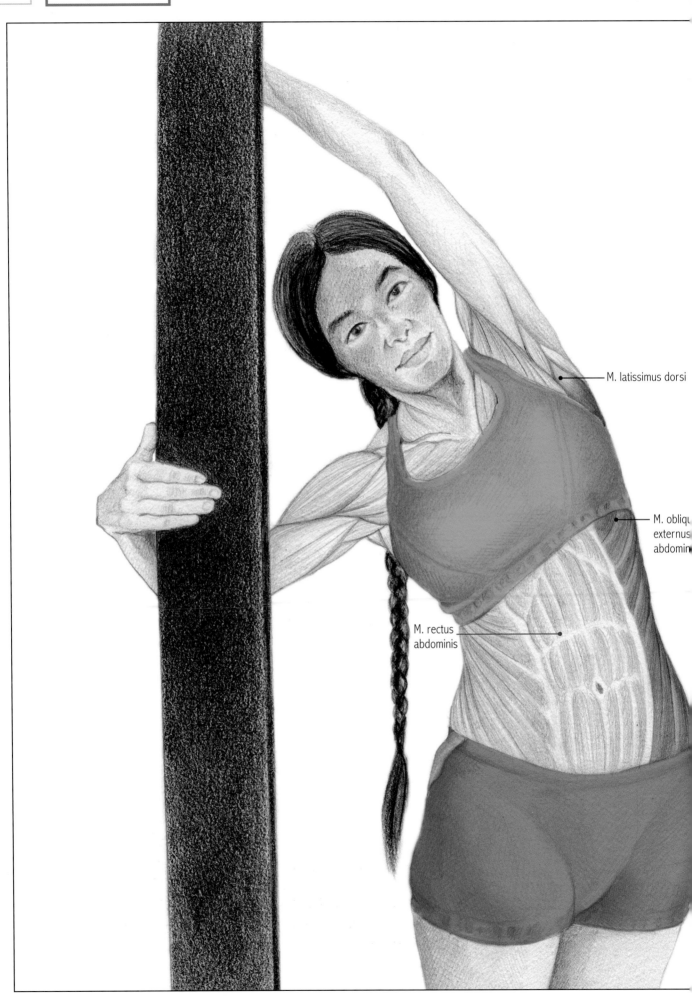

M. latissimus dorsi

M. obliqu
externus
abdomin

M. rectus
abdominis

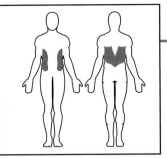

Muscles involved

Principal: Abdominal obliques, latissimus dorsi, quadratus lumborum

Secondary: Transversus abdominus, rectus abdominus

Execution

We position ourselves laterally next to a column or some other similar support with the whole body against the support (especially the foot closest to it). Hold on with the hand that is farther away, above the head, and with the closer hand we hold the support at the level of the waist. Then let yourself fall away laterally, feeling the body arch and feeling the stretch all along this side.

Comments

As with the previous exercise, the force of gravity is enough during this exercise to produce the stretch, and there is no need to force it past its natural movement. As is obvious, once one side has been stretched, switch sides and repeat the exercise for the opposite side.

In addition to stretching the abdominal obliques, it is important to also feel the stretch in the rest of the lateral structures indicated, such as the quadratus lumborum and the transverse abdominus.

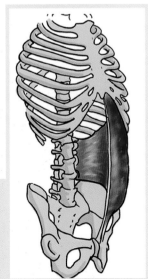

 Although the rectus abdominus, with its unique "board-like" appearance due to its slabs of muscle, is the best-known muscle of the abdomen, what is true is that the abdominal muscles extend throughout the entire waist. When they are healthy and have good muscle tone, they are the perfect natural girdle.

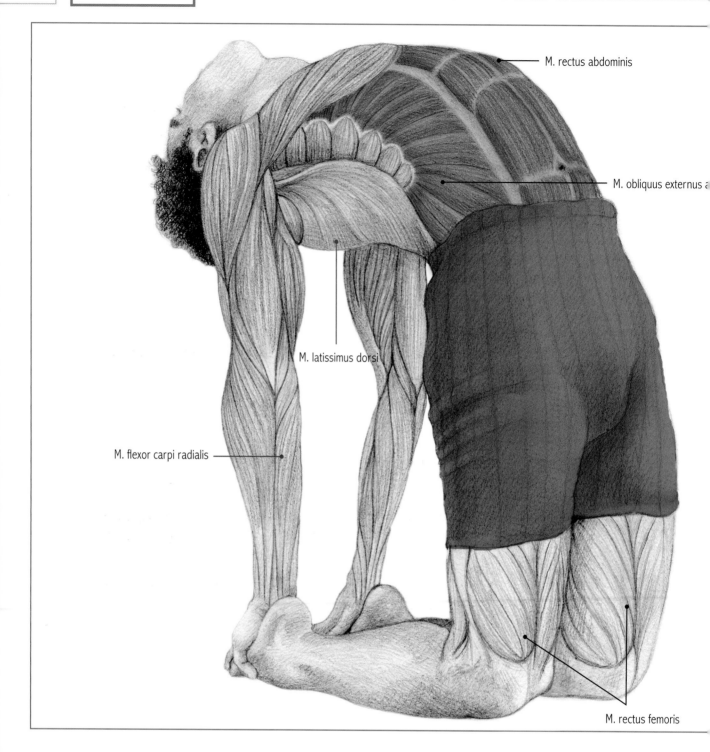

M. rectus abdominis

M. obliquus externus a

M. latissimus dorsi

M. flexor carpi radialis

M. rectus femoris

Variations   4.2... Bridge

This classic exercise which is common to gymnastics and even childrens' games, provides a great stretch of the abdominal area, but in addition to being uncomfortable, it is also not so decisive. There are more comfortable and effective variations explained throughout this book. This exercise starts from the decubitus supine position (laying flat on your back), and then you place your hands and feet firmly on the ground and push the trunk upward. The bottoms of the feet must remain firmly in place and the hands should be pointing toward the feet.

An intermediate step to the final posture of the bridge involves supporting, in principle, the forehead against the ground. Once that position has been mastered, one can move on to the bridge itself. But before performing this posture, one must be conscious of the potential of each person to withstand the stress that the neck is being subjected to.

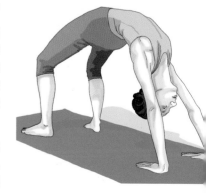

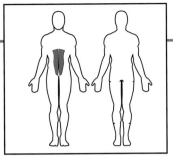

Muscles involved

Principal: Rectus abdominus and the rest of the abdominal muscle group

Secondary: Illiopsoas, rectus femoris, latissimus dorsi, hand flexors

Execution

Down on your knees, with the rest of the body straight, lean backwards little by little (extending the hip) and arching the body until you can touch the ground or your heels.

Comments

This exercise can be somewhat uncomfortable and can cause certain pain in the lower back. For these reasons, it is not very common and can be substituted by any of the other exercises that are described in this book that also stretch the abdomen.

We should remember that not only the muscles are stretched during these exercises; in this exercise, for example, the common anterior vertebral ligament is also stretched.

4.3... Arch

To follow in the line of the uncomfortable and not-recommended exercises, we find this one. Starting from the decubitus prone position (lying face down), you grab your ankles from behind and pull strongly with the arms at the same time that you try to extend the legs, in order to achieve the characteristic "arch." The lumbar tension makes this not recommended, and only some gymnasts should practice it due to the specific demands of their sport.

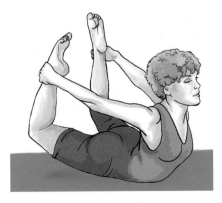

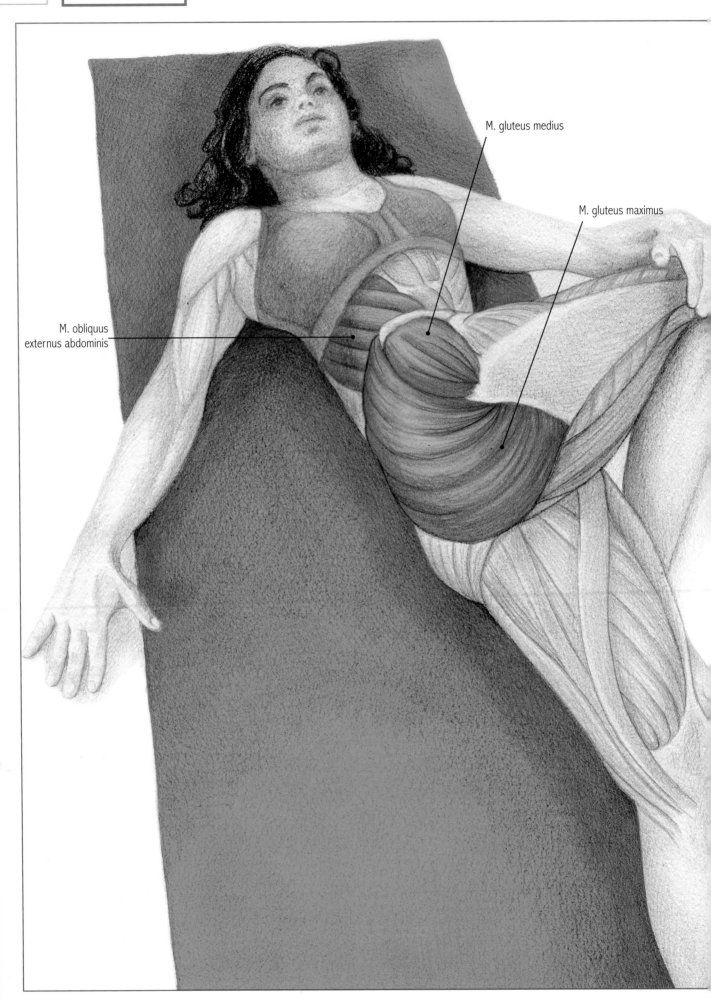

M. gluteus medius

M. gluteus maximus

M. obliquus externus abdominis

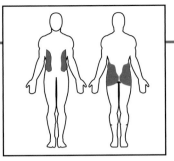

Muscles involved

Principal: Abdominal obliques, gluteus maximus and medius

Secondary: Pyramidal, gemini, obturator internus and obturator externus

Execution

Starting from the decubitus supine position (lying on your back), raise one leg with the knee partly flexed and take it to the opposite side, with the help of the hand on the opposite side to the leg being stretched. With that hand, pull downward on the knee. The rest of the body should remain as still as possible. As a reference, the non-working hand will always remain on the ground. If the flexibility is good and the technique is correct, the shoulder on this side should not have to lift off the ground. The head faces the side opposite to the turn, in order to help maintain the clavicle immobile.

Comments

In this exercise, depending on whether we emphasize the turning of the leg or if we also emphasize the turning of the hip, we will stretch the gluteal area and also the abdominal obliques.

The knee of the leg being lifted should not be extended because this would also put stress on the ischiotibial muscles, while we want the emphasis to be on the muscles of the hip. This includes not only the abdominal obliques, but also the lumbar muscles, which will experience a significant load here.

It is preferable to change sides with every repetition and not do them all to one side before changing over. We should not forget that exercises such as this one not only stretch the large muscle groups of the hip, but also a variety of small muscles and ligaments, which are part of the columnar structure.

Variation   **5.2... With both legs**

The exercise is very similar, except that now, both legs are moved at the same time to the same side. The hand from the target side will assist first in the movement and then in holding the knees in their final position. The rotation must be performed in a very slow and controlled manner, since the weight of the legs falling, without control, could cause too sharp a turn for the column.

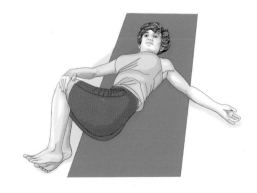

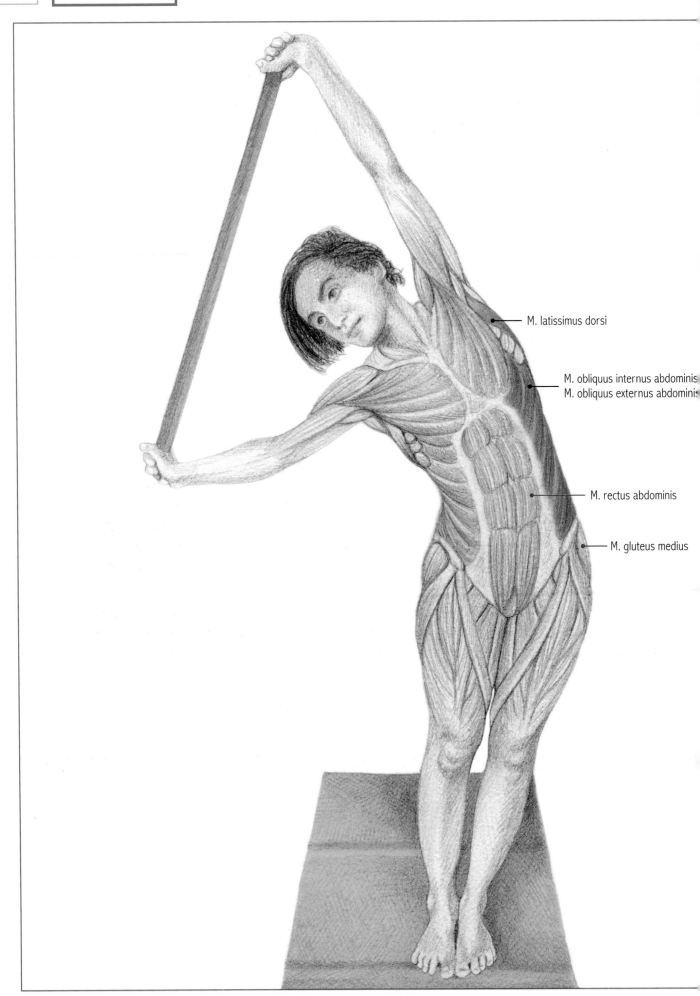

M. latissimus dorsi

M. obliquus internus abdominis
M. obliquus externus abdominis

M. rectus abdominis

M. gluteus medius

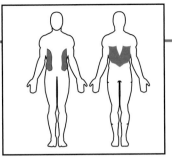

Muscles involved

Principal: Abdominal obliques, latissimus dorsi, quadratus lumborum

Secondary: Transverse abdominus, rectus abdominus, gluteus medius

Execution

Stand in front of a mirror and hold a wooden bar, or something similar, over your head, with the arms extended, and bend laterally up to the point of maximum stretch. The feet will remain slightly apart in order to keep your balance.

Comments

The wooden bar is only a reference to help us maintain the correct posture; this exercise can be performed without a bar as well. The most common mistake is to flex the trunk slightly in an attempt to reach farther down, and the bar makes us keep in mind that the bending should be laterally. The tension will be felt along the entire side of the trunk, from the abdominals to the latissimus dorsi. Precisely in order to achieve all this stretching, the hand from the opposite side should be pointed upward and to the side, so it is not enough to simply raise the arm, but rather to have it actively participate in the exercise.

Once you have reached the final position, you might be able to gain an extra centimeter by completely blowing all the air out of your lungs. Similarly, a point of greater intensity can be achieved by allowing the pelvis to balance out toward the side opposite the stretch, reinforcing the curvature of the body.

Variation	6.2... Variation without a bar

The exact same exercise can also be performed without the aid of a bar, and it is more comfortable if you raise the hand from the side being stretched, while the other hand remains at the waist helping to guard the degree to which the body falls.

In this way, the opposite side will simply stretch passively (there is no need to "hold" the trunk, something which could occur in the exercise with a bar).

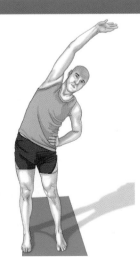

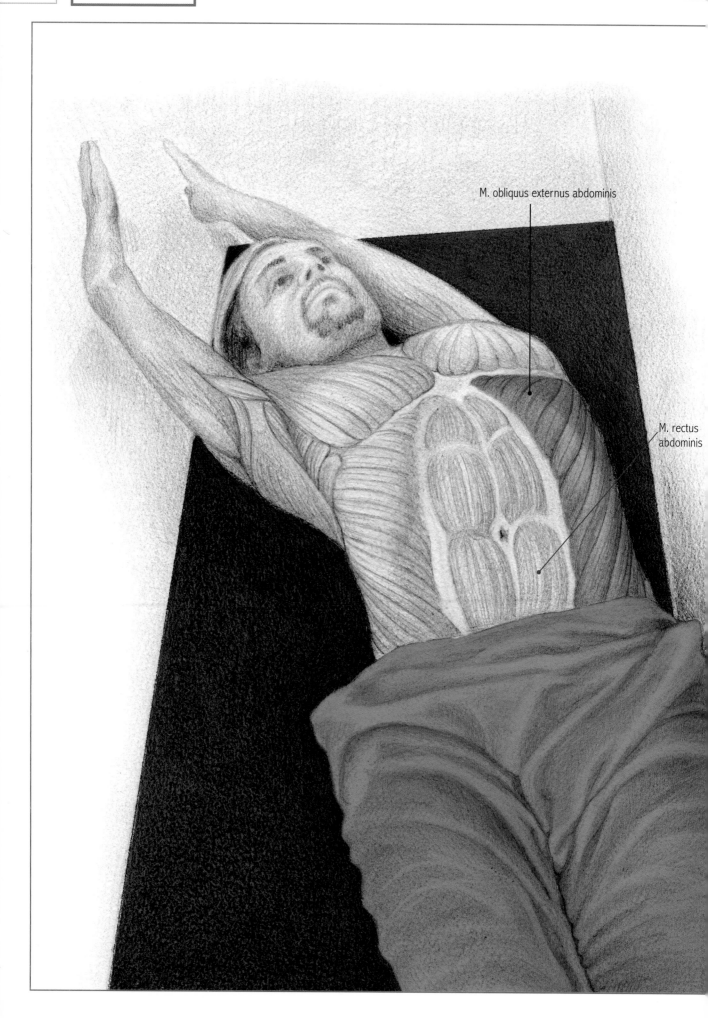

M. obliquus externus abdominis

M. rectus abdominis

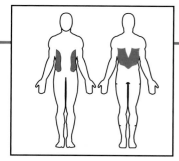

Muscles involved

Principal: Abdominal obliques, latissimus dorsi, quadratus lumborum

Secondary: Transverse abdominus, rectus abdominus, gluteus medius

Execution

Starting from a decubitus supine position (lying on your back) with one whole side of the body supported against a wall, bend toward the opposite side without pulling either the legs or hip away from the wall.

Comments

If you also raise the hand from the area being stretched, you will involve the latissimus dorsi and the teres major muscles, and if you don't, the stretch will be focused on the abdomen. The wall is only a reference so that the legs and the hip can remain immobile during the exercise, something which is not always done when this same movement is performed standing up (see exercise 6). The leg on the side toward which we are stretching can be abducted, bringing it closer to the arm. Once the movement has been completed, it's good to breathe all the air out of the lungs and thereby achive one or more degrees of stretch.

The variation that is performed in the decubitus prone position (lying face down) is equally as valid. Both variations have the advantage of eliminating the bothersome component of balance that is present when we perform the exercise standing up.

 Postural scoliosis (the lateral deviation of the spinal column due to poor posture) improves enormously with a combination of three elements: optimizing the posture (specially while sitting), stretching the side that is shortened, and strengthening the opposite side. As in many other cases, it is a compensated scoliosis (lateral curve and counter-curve), and it is difficult to establish very specific exercises. Only global strength and flexibility exercises can be performed, although they will also provide improvement (in addition to the physiotherapy treatments).

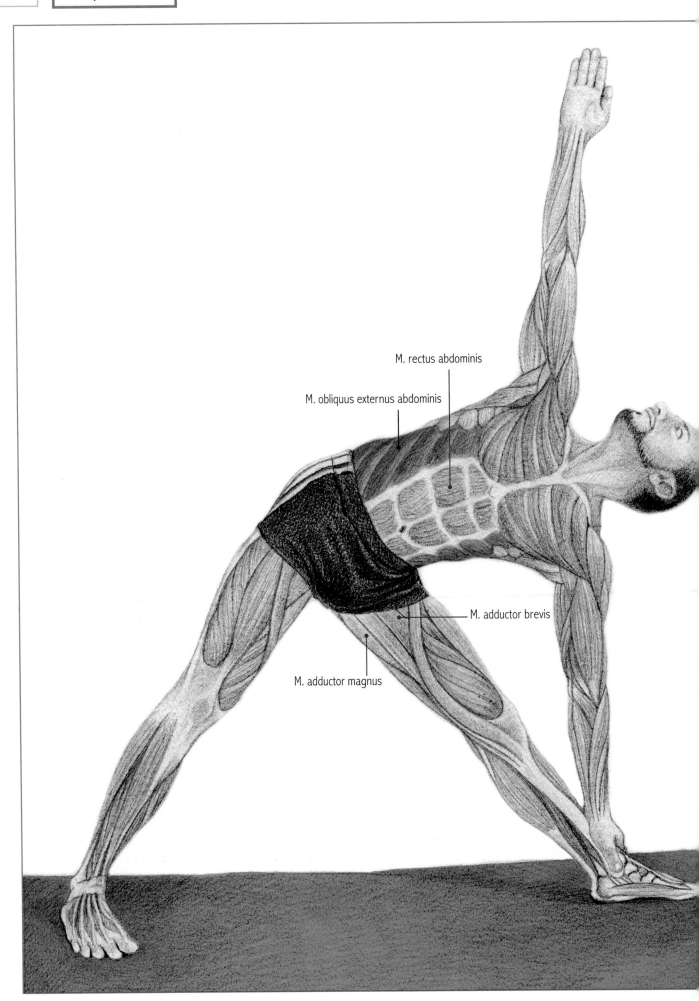

M. rectus abdominis

M. obliquus externus abdominis

M. adductor brevis

M. adductor magnus

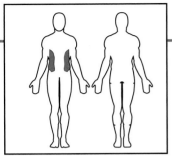

Muscles involved

Principal: Abdominal obliques

Secondary: Transverse abdominus, rectus abdominus, gluteus medius, adductors

Execution

Starting from a standing position, facing a mirror, open the legs moderately and bend the torso laterally. At the same time, raise the arm (abduction) of the side being stretched.

Comments

In this exercise, otherwise similar to the ones previously explained, there is the slight difference of the stretching of the gluteus medius and, secondarily, the adductors. Otherwise, it does not provide any significant advantages over the other exercises.

 Although the majority of stretching exercises require that the respiration be natural and paused, there is one technique that will add a greater degree of stretch to some exercises. It involves taking in a deep breath without altering your posture, and then exhaling completely at the same time that you try to stretch the area a little bit more. This technique, which can only be held for a few seconds, is effective in the movements that affect the thoracic cavity and the vertebral column, since when you empty the lungs, you achieve greater mobility of the trunk.

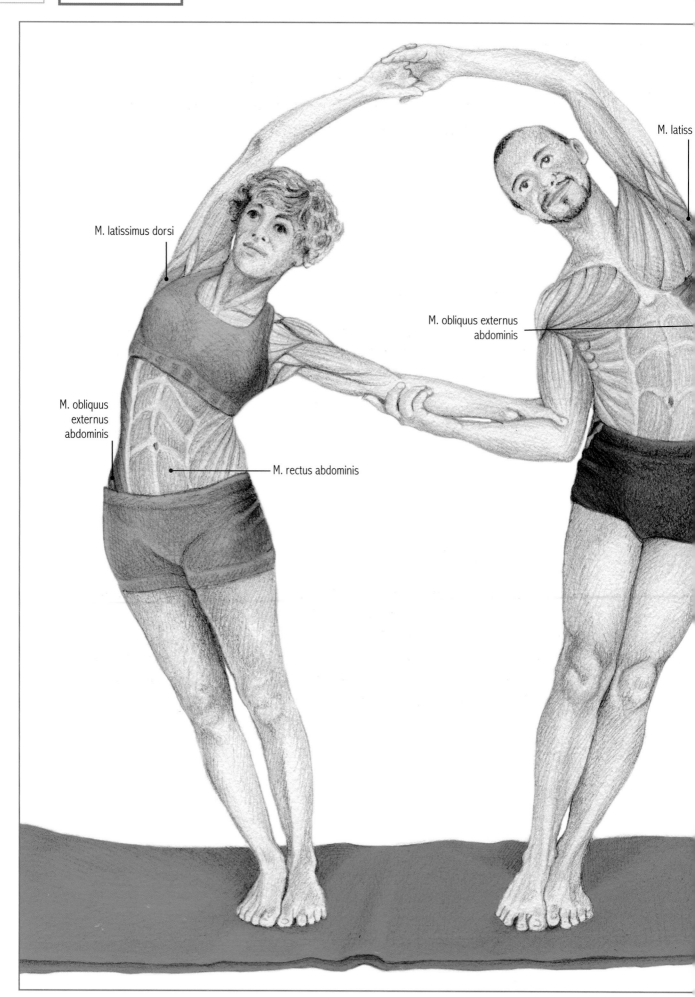

M. latiss

M. latissimus dorsi

M. obliquus externus abdominis

M. obliquus externus abdominis

M. rectus abdominis

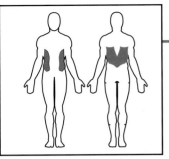

Muscles involved

Principal: Abdominal obliques, latissimus dorsi, quadratus lumborum

Secondary: Transverse abdominus, rectus abdominus

Execution

Stand side by side with your training partner in front of a mirror, but with enough separation between you so as to reach each other with the arms. Mutually hold each other's forearm on the closer side, and your hands of the other side above the head. From there, let yourself gently fall away from your training partner.

Comments

In this exercise, it is preferable that the training partners be of a similar height and weight. Otherwise, the posture will be too uncomfortable and much less effective. The idea is to achieve a stretch of the entire lateral area (gluteus medius, obliques, latissimus dorsi).

The exercises performed with a training partner are not always better than those performed individually. Although the component of motivation tends to be greater when one trains with a partner, you can access that motivation simply by training alongside each other.

 Although training with someone of the same height and weight can be preferable in some stretching exercises, the decisive factor is doing it with some who has the same objectives and the same determination in achieving them as you do.

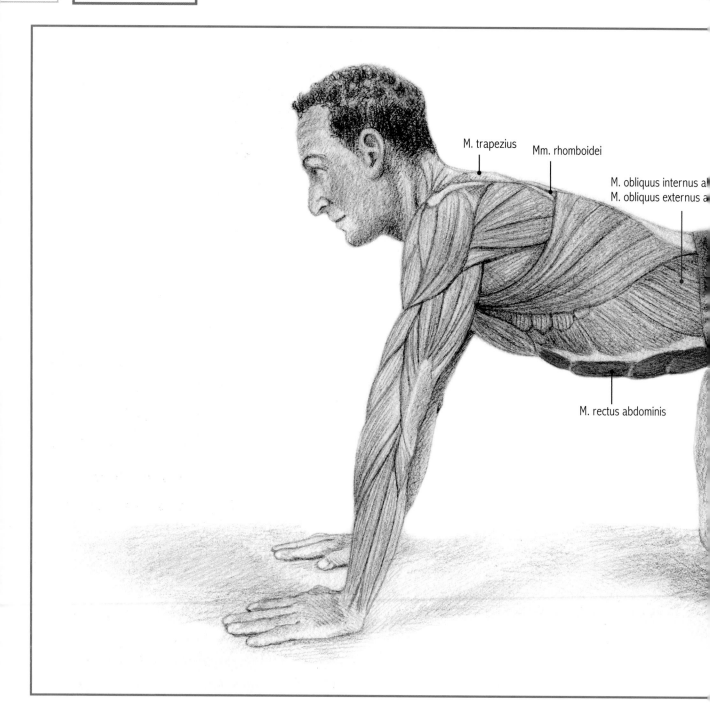

M. trapezius   Mm. rhomboidei

M. obliquus internus a▮
M. obliquus externus a▮

M. rectus abdominis

Comments

This simple exercise can be classified under exercises for mobility of the spinal column and the sm▮ muscles that surround it. The "hug" to the legs can be done from under the legs (as the image shows) from above them, following the flexion of the knees. What is important is to distend the vertebral colum▮ especially in the lumbar region.

The position must allow the balancing of the body along the entire posterior surface of the trunk.

There is one variation in which this posture is taken to the extreme, totally elevating the lumbar regio▮ touching the ground behind the head with your feet. The problem with this exercise is the cervical are▮ subjected to an excessive flexion at the same time that it has to support a large portion of the bodyweig▮

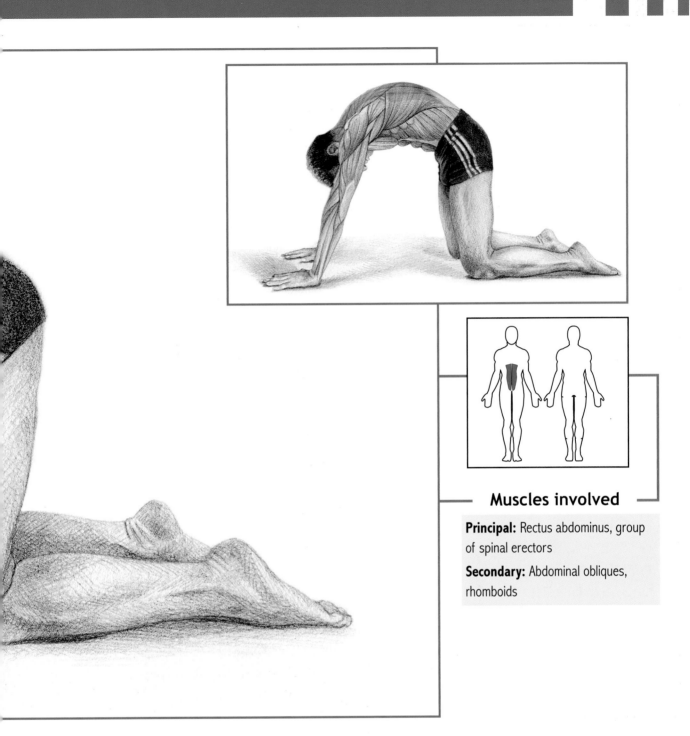

Muscles involved

Principal: Rectus abdominus, group of spinal erectors

Secondary: Abdominal obliques, rhomboids

Execution

From a quadruped starting position (on your hands and knees), contract the abdomen in order to curve the spine; and from that position, relax and press the torso down in order to create the opposite curvature. Take a deep breath and extend the abdomen, then exhale to contract it.

 In almost all stretching exercises that are performed on the ground, it is imperative to have a padded surface on which to do them. A simple support on an inappropriate ground could lead to an injury. Individual exercise mats are available on the market, such as the ones used in camping tents, which may be useful. In addition, one should cover the mat with a towel in order to prevent the discomfort caused by excessive sweat on the mat.

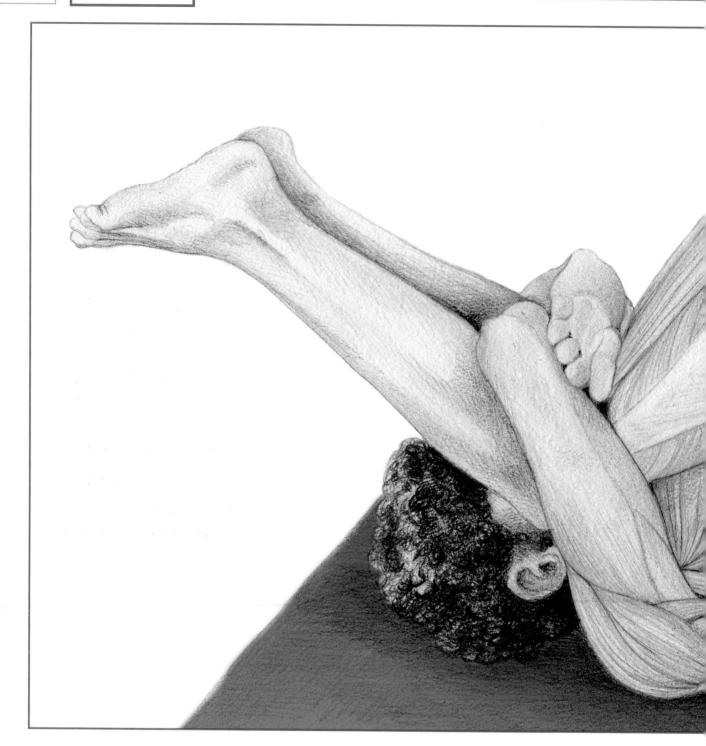

Comments

Due to the tension of the rotator muscles of the trunk, this exercise could not be performed effectiv[e] without the help of another person. In fact, the person performing the stretch must relax the abdomi[nal] area and exhale during the turn so that the training partner can do his work correctly. In case the help [of] a partner is not available, one may place the hands behind the head and perform the exercise by himse[lf].

The legs should press against the bench (closing in adduction), to be able to hold the hip in place. If t[he] person performing the stretch sat on a bench in a different way than is described here, it would pro[ve] very difficult for him or her to immobilize the hip area. You should not make the mistake of resting t[he] wooden bar across the back of the neck; the correct form is to rest it on the back of the shoulders and t[he] trapezius muscle. On the other hand, you should try to have the entire vertebral column perform the twi[st] not just the upper portion.

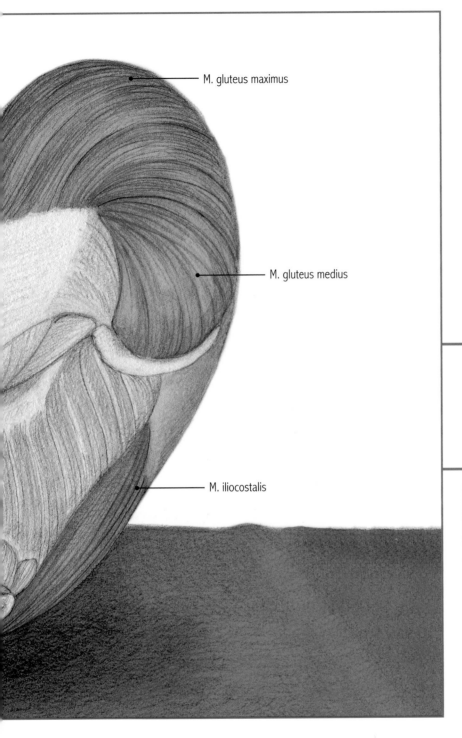

M. gluteus maximus

M. gluteus medius

M. iliocostalis

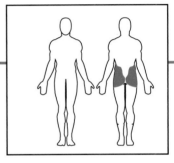

Muscles involved

Principal: Abdominal obliques

Secondary: Transverse abdominus, quadratus lumborum

Execution

Seated on a flat bench (or straddling a flat bench as if you were riding a horse), without a back support, hold on to a wooden bar (or something similar) across the shoulders. The training partner stands behind you in order to hold on to the bar, and slowly turn the trunk to one of the sides until the maximum tension necessary is felt, relax to the front before repeating to the opposite side.

 A bad posture when sitting, which eliminates the natural lumbar curvature, places all the bodyweight upon the coccyx. It is more appropriate to sit over the ischial bones, and especially over the strong and thick gluteus maximus. Keeping in mind that many people spend one-third of their lives sitting, we should think about whether we are doing it correctly.

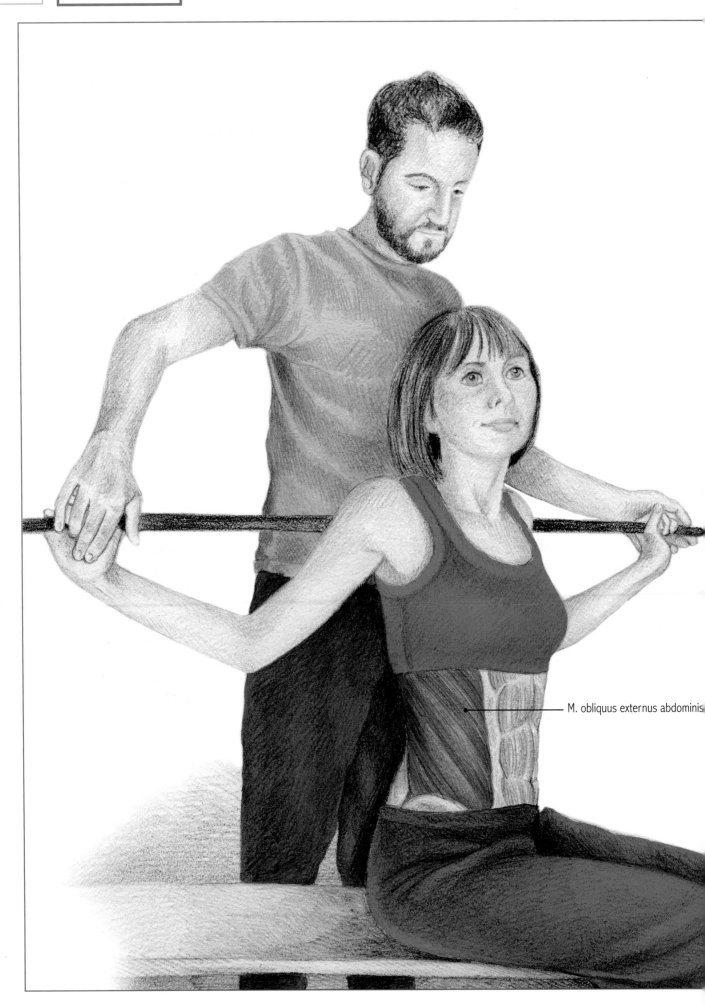

M. obliquus externus abdominis

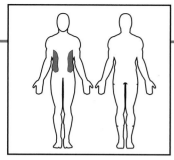

Muscles involved

Principal: Abdominal obliques

Secondary: Transverse abdominus, quadratus lumborum

Execution

Seated on a flat bench (or straddling a flat bench as if you were riding a horse), without a back support, hold on to a wooden bar (or something similar) across the shoulders. The training partner stands behind you in order to hold on to the bar and slowly turn the trunk to one of the sides until the maximum tension necessary is felt. Relax to the front before repeating on the opposite side.

Comments

Due to the tension of the rotator muscles of the trunk, this exercise could not be performed effectively without the help of another person. In fact, the person performing the stretch must relax the abdominal area and exhale during the turn so that the training partner can do his work correctly. In case the help of a partner is not available, one may place the hands behind the head and perform the exercise by himself.

The legs should press against the bench (closing in adduction) to be able to hold the hip in place. If the person performing the stretch sat on a bench in a different way than is described here, it would prove very difficult for him or her to immobilize the hip area. You should not make the mistake of resting the wooden bar across the back of the neck; the correct form is to rest it on the back of the shoulders and the trapezius muscle. On the other hand, you should try to have the entire vertebral column perform the twist, not just the upper portion.

 A bad posture when sitting, which eliminates the natural lumbar curvature, places all the body weight upon the coccyx. It is more appropriate to sit over the ischial bones, and especially over the strong and thick gluteus maximus. Keeping in mind that many people spend one-third of their lives sitting, we should think about whether we are doing it correctly.

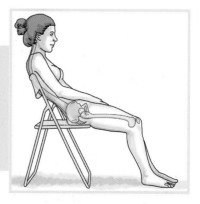

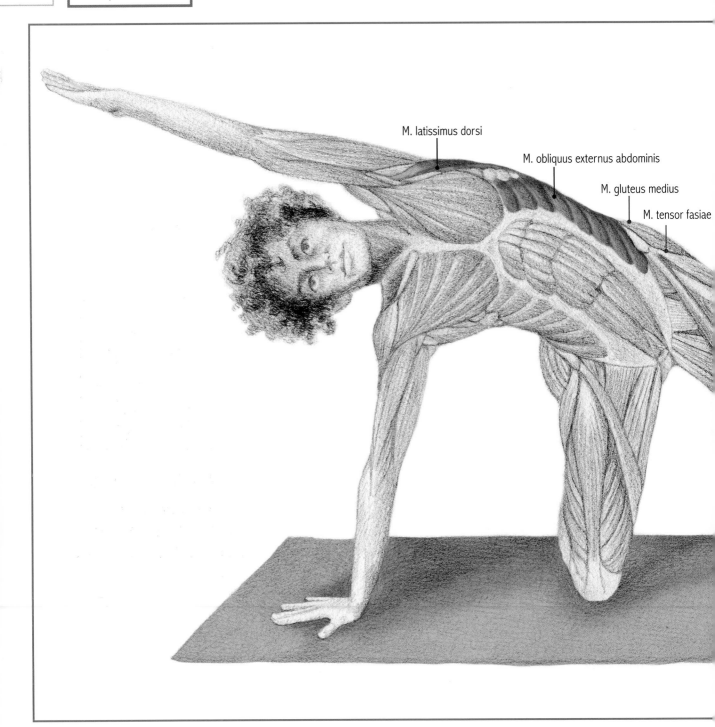

M. latissimus dorsi

M. obliquus externus abdominis

M. gluteus medius

M. tensor fasiae

Execution

Begin by sitting on your heels (on a padded mat). From there, one leg is extended to the side (in abduction) whi the ipsilateral arm is raised. The opposite hand is placed on the ground to the side. Finally, the raised arm is take to its maximum lateral extension, as is shown in the picture.

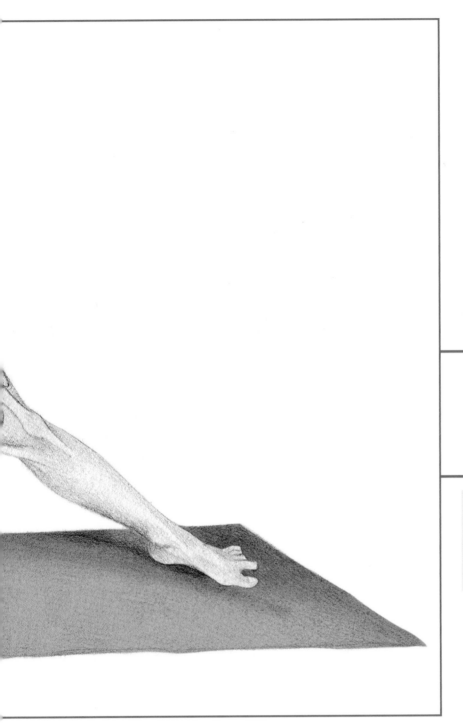

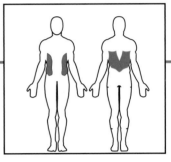

Muscles involved

Principal: Abdominal obliques, latissimus dorsi, quadratus lumborum

Secondary: Gluteus medius, tensor fascia lata

Comments

As in the equivalent exercises that were performed standing up (see exercises 6 and 8), the stretch should be felt all along the side of the body; to help us achieve this feeling, it may be useful to try to separate as much as possible the hand and the foot from the side that is being stretched.

 Is yoga the perfect means for performing stretches correctly? Unfortunately, no. But that does not mean that it is not an adequate philosophy on physical exercise, but rather that not all yoga exercises are healthy, and there are exceptions, such as the ones that have been described throughout this book. Similarly, not all stretches as they have traditionally been practiced in the world of sports are recommended.

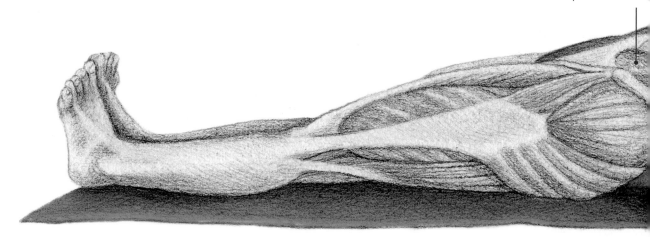

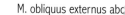

M. obliquus externus abd

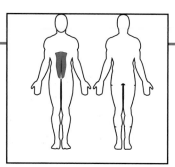

Muscles involved

Principal: Rectus abdominus

Secondary: Abdominal obliques (major and minor), transversus abdominus, latissimus dorsi

---

Execution

A padded mat is placed on the ground (a towel or a rolled-up gymnastics mat are also useful), and y lie down on our back on top of the mat in such a way that the padded support is located underneath t lumbar region (under the lower back). From that starting position, extend the arms over the head and t to stretch as much as possible.

rectus abdominis

M. latissimus dorsi

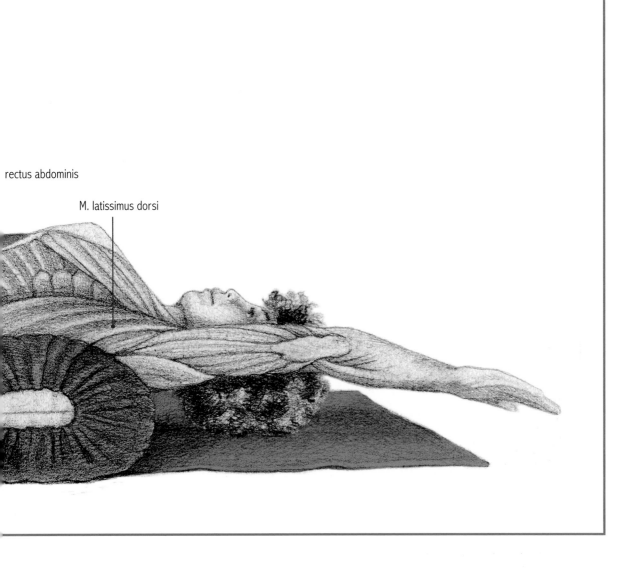

Comments

This simple exercise is appropriate for those people who suffer from posture-related pain of the muscles of the spinal column. The only precaution is that the padding must be adequate, since one that is too high and/or too hard could be uncomfortable, and the exact opposite would be quite ineffective. This is a stretch that, because of its simplicity and comfort, can be performed by people who have difficulties with movement as well as by the elderly.

The variation that is performed without the padding can also be done, but in this case the objective is to be able to maintain the lower back firmly pressed against the ground, followed by relaxation. The posture for this variation should be with the legs flexed and the bottoms of the feet planted on the floor; from that position, press the lumbar region downward and relax it after a few seconds.

 Sometimes, we are only conscious of the importance of the lower back muscles after we experience pain. In these cases, something as simple as lifting the arms in front of us can cause a sharp pain in the lower back. But it is not only that, this same gesture means that the pressure on our feet is displaced toward the toes (and we have thus modified the body`s center of gravity). This illustrates how all the areas of the body are kept in a constant equilibrium of tension-relaxation, and that there is a true connection between them.

Appendix 1

TEST FOR EVALUATING MOBILITY

Although everyone has a general idea of their overall physical condition and of their ability to stretch, in particular, the following tests will help to statistically place your level and evaluate progress. They are not listed here to evaluate the flexibility of the entire body; their purpose is to estimate in a general way, the person's degree of mobility, and that is the reason why they focus on the two most mobile joints in the human body — the hip and the shoulder.

HOW TO PERFORM THE TESTS

The proper way to perform these tests would be to do some warm-up exercises in order to achieve good results without risking injury. The tests should be performed by following the instructions provided for each one. Some will differ by age and gender, whereas others are appropriate for all people.

There is no reason to perform any of these tests if you are exhausted or injured since they are designed to be performed by healthy adults.

HOW TO INTERPRET THE RESULTS

The tables have been developed thanks to the measurements obtained from hundreds of subjects, which make possible the development of statistical tables. The person performing the test could compare his or her results with the average. That is, if the person's results approach 100, he or she will have an excellent level of flexibility for the area measured; if the results correspond to the middle portion of the table, that means that he or she is about average, and so on.

The most accurate way to make an evaluation is to use different tests and divide the results between the number of tests performed. Three attempts are allowed for each test, and only the best result is counted. For example,

On the first test, perform three tries and record the best result in the following way:

You obtain 39, 40 and 39, so record 40 points. Do the same with the subsequent tests.

1. You perform three tests, and get the following results: 40, 55 and 70 points.

2. Add: 40 + 55 + 70 = 165 points.

3. Divide the result by the number of tests performed: 165 / 3 = 55 points.

4. The overall result of the test is "55 points," and in this case, it is right about average. Also think of the points as representing an average, that is, 55%.

Test of Flexibility

Deep flexion with legs flexed

1. Stand with bare feet separated slightly more than shoulder-width apart.

2. Place a wooden board or something similar between the feet, in line with the heels.

3. Flex the torso and the legs, passing your arms between your legs, toward the back. Push the wooden board (guiding it, without throwing it) in one continuous motion backward. The push will be made with the tips of the fingers of both hands at the same time, and the movement should be sufficiently controlled so that when you reach the furthermost point toward the back, the board remains in touch with the fingertips.

4. Measure the distance between the initial placement of the board (the heels of your feet) and the final position reached.

5. You will get three attempts, recording the best one of the three. The following table shows the results between 10 and 55 centimeters of displacement of the board, independently of gender.

Men and women		Men and women	
cm	points	cm	points
10	1	33	52
11	3	34	54
12	5	35	56
13	7	36	58
14	10	37	61
15	12	38	63
16	14	39	65
17	16	40	67
18	18	41	70
19	21	42	72
20	23	43	74
21	25	44	76
22	27	45	78
23	30	46	81
24	32	47	83
25	34	48	85
26	36	49	87
27	38	50	90
28	41	51	92
29	43	52	94
30	45	53	96
31	47	54	98
32	50	55	100

Source: Ballesteros, Legido and Segovia (96))

Deep flexion with legs straight

1. Stand with your feet bare approximately shoulder-width apart, on a stand approximately 20 cm off the ground.

2. Without bending the knees, flex the trunk bringing your fingers toward the ground.

3. Measure the distance from the ground (not from the stand) to the fingertips.

4. Repeat the exercise three times, recording the best result. The following table shows the results between 10 and 50 cm for men, and between 0 and 40 cm for women.

Men		Women	
cm	points	cm	points
50	1	40	1
49	3	39	3
48	6	38	6
47	8	37	8
46	11	36	11
45	13	35	13
44	16	34	16
43	18	33	18
42	21	32	21
41	23	31	23
40	26	30	26
39	28	29	28
38	31	28	31
37	33	27	33
36	36	26	36
35	38	25	38
24	41	24	41
33	43	23	43
32	46	22	46
31	48	21	48
30	51	20	51
29	53	19	53
28	56	18	56
27	58	17	58
26	61	16	61
25	63	15	63
24	66	14	66
23	68	13	68
22	71	12	71
21	73	11	73
20	76	10	76
19	78	9	78
18	81	8	81
17	83	7	83
16	86	6	86
15	88	5	88
14	91	4	91
13	93	3	93
12	96	2	96
11	98	1	98
10	100	0	100

Source: Ballesteros, Legido and Segovia (96)

Flexion – extension of the shoulders

1. Hold a wooden bar or something similar with a pronated grip in front of the body, over the thighs. Keep the hands and feet shoulder-width apart.

2. Elevate, by flexing the shoulders and the wooden bar over the head, and lower it behind the shoulders toward the glutes.

3. With each successive attempt, widen your grip upon the wooden bar.

4. When you finally manage to complete the range of motion, record the width of the grip on the bar.

5. The value, valid for both sexes, is the width of the grip on the bar minus the width of the shoulders.

Men and women		Men and women	
value	points	value	points
100	1	75	51
99	3	74	53
98	5	73	55
97	7	72	57
96	9	71	59
95	11	70	61
94	13	69	63
93	15	68	65
92	17	67	67
91	19	66	69
90	21	65	71
89	23	64	73
88	25	63	75
87	27	62	77
86	29	61	79
85	31	60	81
84	33	59	83
83	35	58	85
82	37	57	87
81	39	56	89
80	41	55	91
79	43	54	93
78	45	53	95
77	47	52	97
76	49	51	99
		50	100

Source: Ballesteros, Legido and Segovia (96)

Shoulder mobility

1. Standing or seated, lift one arm over the head and flex the elbow of the other behind the trunk.

2. Try touching the tips of the fingers of both hands behind the back.

3. Record the value in centimeters. The table shows the measurements between 0 and 24 cm. When it is possible to place the fingers of one hand over those of the other, it is considered a score <1 (100 points).

Men and women		Men and women	
value	points	value	points
>24	0	12	52
24	4	11	56
23	8	10	60
22	12	9	64
21	16	8	68
20	20	7	72
19	24	6	76
18	28	5	80
17	32	4	84
16	36	3	88
15	40	2	92
14	44	1	96
13	48	<1	100

Source: Ballesteros, Legido and Segovia (96)

Bibliography used for the tests

Ballesteros, J.M., Legido, J.C. and Segovia, J.C. (1996): "Evaluation of physical condition through the test". Ed. Ediciones Pedagógicas. Madrid

García, J.M., Navarro, M and Ruiz, J.A. (1996): "Tests for the evaluation of motor capacity in sports".

Ed. Gymnos (Madrid)

Appendix 2

Movements and the Principal and Secondary Muscles Involved in Each Joint

SHOULDER

Abduction: Middle, front and rear deltoids, supraspinatus, biceps brachii (long head). After approx. 90°; serratus anterior, trapezius

Horizontal abduction: Rear deltoids

Adduction: Latissimus dorsi, teres major, pectoralis major, triceps brachii (long head), biceps brachii (short head), deltoids (clavicular and spinal), coracobrachialis

Horizontal adduction: Pectoralis major, front deltoid, coracobrachialis

Flexion: Front deltoids, coracobrachialis, biceps brachii (long head), pectoralis major (clavicular), serratus anterior

Extension: Latissimus dorsi, rear deltoids, teres major, triceps brachii (long head), pectoralis major (from 90° of flexion)

External/lateral rotation: Infraspinatus, rear deltoids, teres minor

Internal/medial rotation: Subscapularis, pectoralis major, front deltoids, latissimus dorsi, teres major

ELBOW

Flexion: Biceps brachii, brachialis anterior, brachioradialis, extensor carpi radialis longus, pronator teres, palmaris longus, flexor carpi radialis, flexor carpi ulnaris

Extension: Triceps brachii, anconeus

FOREARM AND HAND

Wrist flexion: Flexor digitorum longus superficialis and profundus. Flexor carpi radialis/palmaris major, flexor carpi ulnaris, palmaris longus, flexor pollicis longus

Wrist extension: Extensor digitorum longus, extensor carpi radialis longus and extensor carpi radialis brevis, extensor pollicis longus

Supination: Biceps brachii, brachioradialis (from pronation), short supinator, abductor pollicis longus, extensor pollicis longus, extensor carpi radialis (on occasion)

Pronation: Pronator teres, pronator quadratus, brachioradialis (from supination), palmaris major/ flexor carpi radialis, extensor carpi radialis longus

Radial flexion/abduction of the wrist: Extensor carpi radialis longus and brevis, abductor and extensor pollicis longus, flexor carpi radialis, flexor pollicis longus

Ulnar flexion / abduction of the wrist: Extensor and flexor carpi ulnaris. Extensor digitorum

HIP

Abduction: Gluteus medius, minimus and maximus (superficial), tensor fascia lata, sartorius, piriformis, obturator internus

Adduction: Adductor major longus and brevis (and minimus, when it exists), gracilis, pectineus, illiopsoas, gluteus maximus, quadratus femoris, obturator externus, semitendinosus

Flexion: Illiopsoas, quadriceps (rectus femoris), biceps femoris (long head), gluteus medius, adductor major (posterior), piriformis

External/lateral rotation: Gluteus major, quadratus femoris, gluteus medius (posterior), obturator internus, illiopsoas, biceps femoris (long head), adductor major, sartorius, piriformis

Internal/medial rotation: Semitendinosus, semimembranosus, gluteus minimus, tensor fascia lata, adductor major (in part), pectineus (when there is abduction of the hip) gluteus medius (ocassionally, its anterior fibers)

KNEE

Extension: Quadriceps, gluteus maximus (superficial, together with tensor fascia lata)

Flexion: Semimembranosus, semitendinosus and biceps femoris, gracilis, gastrocnemius, sartorius, popliteus, tensor fascia lata (according to some studies)

External rotation: Biceps femoris, slight contribution from tensor fascia lata

Internal rotation: Semimembranosus and semitendinosus, gracilis, popliteus, sartorius

ANKLE AND FOOT

Dorsal flexion: Tibialis anterior, extensor digitorum longus, peroneus, extensor hallucis longus

Plantar flexion: Gastrocnemius, soleus, peroneus longus and brevis, flexor digitorum longus, tibialis posterior, flexor hallucis longus

Appendix 3

Standard Degrees of Mobility [1]

The following data are the degrees of mobility standardized according to measurements in hundreds of subjects. Differing from these values does not necessarily imply a pathology; for example, people with significant muscle masses have less mobility for the simple reason that said muscles masses meet and prevent further flexion.

SHOULDER

Abduction: 60° pure (scapulo – humeral), and 120° to 180° associated to the rest of the shoulder

Horizontal abduction: 30° (in flexion of the shoulder)

Adduction: 0° (impeded by the body) or 30° to 45° in slight flexion of the shoulder

Horizontal adduction: (in flexion of the shoulder) 140°

Flexion: 45° to 90°

Extension: 50°

External / lateral rotation: 80°

Internal / medial rotation: 30°

ELBOW

Flexion: 145° active, 160° passive

Extension: 0°

FOREARM AND WRIST

Wrist flexion: 85°

Wrist extension: 85°

Supination: 90°

Pronation: 85°

Radial flexion/wrist abduction: 15°

Ulnar flexion/wrist adduction: approximately 50°

Source: Kapandji, A.I. (1998): "Joint physiology". Ed. Maloine (Paris)

HIP

Abduction: 30° to 180°

Adduction: 0° to 30° if accompanied by flexion or extension

Flexion: 90° with the knee extended to 145° if the knee is flexed

Extension: 20° with the knee extended to 10° if the knee is flexed

External/lateral rotation: 60°

Internal/medial rotation: 35°

KNEE

Extension: 0°

Flexion: 140° to 160° depending on whether it is active or passive tension

External rotation: 40°

Internal rotation: 30°

ANKLE AND FOOT

Dorsal flexion: 30°

Plantar flexion: 50°

Appendix 4

Dictionary of Terms Used

The following terms are necessary to understand the explanations given throughout this book. Some of the definitions have been taken from the "Dictionary of the Spanish Language" of the Royal Academy of Spain (RAE), and have been adapted by the author to the subject of this book.

A

Abduction: Movement by which a limb is moved away from the midline, which conceptually divides the body in symmetrical halves. It generally applies to the movement of an arm away from the trunk or of a leg away from the hip

Akinesia: Lack of movement

Adduction: Movement by which a limb is brought toward the midline which conceptually divides the body in symmetrical halves. It generally applies to the movement of an arm toward the trunk or of a leg toward the hip

Agonist: Muscle that performs a movement

Allodynamic: Movement produced by a force that varies along the length of its trajectory. In practice, any human movement is allodynamic

Anatomical: See "position"

Anisometric: Dynamic, having unsymmetrical parts or unequal dimensions or measurements

Antagonist: The muscle opposite to the one performing the movement

Anterior (area): In front, ventral

Apnea: Lack of, or stoppage in, breathing

Atrophy: Decrease in the size of one or more tissues that make up an organ, with the subsequent reduction in volume, weight and functional activity, due to the lack of or delay in the process of nutrition. Especifically with respect to a muscle, it is a direct result of the reduction in physical activity

B

Biomechanics: The science that studies the application of mechanics to living beings (see "mechanics")

C

Center of gravity: Imaginary point that represents the center of the weight of the body or of any object, around which all the other parts are balanced

Circumduction: Compound movement of a joint, like the circular motion of the scapulo-humeral joint (shoulder) or the coccyx-femoral (hip)

Coaptar: Ajustar

Coapt: Fit tightly and fasten; adjust

D

Decubitus prone: Lying face down

Decubitus (supine): Lying on one's back

Direction: Line formed by a point in motion, independently of its target

Distal (area): Removed from the torso; from the origin

Distend: relax or decrease the tension

Dynamic (contraction): see "anisometric"

E

Exercise: Any voluntary motor movement that is intended to work the muscles

Elasticity: The property of a muscle (or other solid parts) to recover their shape and extension once the force that stretched it and deformed it ceases

Elongate: Stretch

Expiration: Exhaling; expelling the air that has been inspired; blowing

Extension: Unfolding of a joint that was previously flexed

F

Fiber: The contractile cell of the muscle

Fibula: The smaller of the two bones of the lower leg

Flexibility: Quality of being flexible, or capacity to bend

Flexion: Action and effect of bending the body or a limb. From the anatomical position, it is the bringing closer of the anterior parts of the body; except in the leg, which is bringing closer from the rear

Force: Strength, robustness, and the capacity to move a weight or resistance. Force = mass x acceleration

H

Heterokinetic: Movement of non-constant speed; in practice, any human movement

Hyperextension: Extension beyond the anatomical position

Horizontal (plane): See "transverse"

Hypertrophy: Increase in the volume of an organ, such as the increase in the size of a muscle

I

Intensity: Percentage of work in relation to the maximum force applied to a muscular effort in particular. Also any variable that makes any exercise quantitatively more difficult

Inspiration: Inhaling air into the lungs

Isodynamic: Movement produced by the same force along the entire trajectory. In practice, it cannot occur with human movements, although it can be approached

Isokinetic: Movement with constant velocity, generally associated with a maximum force, although in practice, it never actually occurs in human movements

Isotonic: Movement in which the same muscle tone is maintained throughout the entire movement; not feasible in athletic activities

J

Joint: Junction of one bone with another; generally mobile

K

Kyphosis: Convex curving of the spine; natural in the upper back

L

Lateral (area): Away from the mid-saggital plane

Lateral decubitus: Position in which a person is lying down on his or her side

Longitudinal (plane): Perpendicular to the ground, that is, the plane that divides the body into an anterior and a posterior region

Lordosis: Curve of posterior concavity; natural in the lumbar and cervical regions

Luxation: Dislocation; that is, when a bone is forced out of its joint

M

Mass: Physical quality that expresses the amount of matter that a body contains. Its unit in the International System is the kilogram (kg). It is usually confused with "weight" though in everyday life, this technical misuse of the terminology is acceptable

Mechanics: Science that studies the equilibrium and movement of bodies subjected to forces (see "biomechanics")

Medial (area): Close to the mid-sagittal plane

Mobility (joint): Range of movement that is limited by the meeting of bones or muscle masses

N

NMR Nuclear Magnetic Resonance: Technique for studying the muscles (among other things) whereby one can compare contrasts in the participation of different muscles in an exercise.

P

Passive (movement): Movement performed without the help of muscle contraction by the person

Perineal: Anatomical space located between the anus and the sexual organs

Phase (concentric/positive): Movement of contraction in muscle shortening

Phase (eccentric/negative): The opposite of concentric or positive

Position (anatomical): Standing up, head straight, legs slightly separated, arms at the sides, and hands supinated (showing the palms)

Posterior (area): Behind, dorsal

Pronation: Movement of the forearm that turns the wrist inward, as when picking an object up from a table

Proximal (area): Close to the torso; to the origin. The opposite of distal

Q

Quadruped: Position in which the hands and feet or knees are placed on the ground

R

Reflex: Involuntary movement in response to a stimulus

Repetition: Complete movement of contraction and relaxation, composed of a concentric and an eccentric phase (positive and negative, respectively)

Rotation: Turn

S

Saggital (plane): Perpendicular to the longitudinal and transverse. That is, the plane that divides the body into two symmetrical halves of right and left.

Series: A set of one or several continuous "repetitions" of a movement, until rest, in a given exercise

Stretching: The activity of performing several stretches.

Supination: Movement of the forearm that turns the hand outward, showing the palm; as if you were taking a bowl of soup to the table

Synnergistic: Term used to designate the other muscle(s) to perform the same action

T

Tear: Referring to the muscle, lack of continuity of the muscle with irregular borders, generally produced from overstretching the muscle

Transverse (plane): Perpendicular to the longitudinal; that is, the plane that divides the body into an upper and lower region

U

Ulna: The medial bone in the forearm

V

Ventilate: To renew the air in the lungs

Ventral: Anterior, frontal

Vertical (plane): see Longitudinal

Index of Exercises

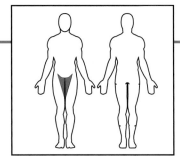

Muscles involved

Principal: Adductors

Secondary: Ischiotibial muscles, gracilis, sartorius, popliteus

Execution

Seated on the ground, preferably with the back resting on a wall (especially beginners), bring the feet together and open the legs in abduction with the knees flexed. From this position, press the knees toward the ground.

Comments

The heels of the feet must remain close to the pelvis. The movements that involve bouncing, taking the knees toward the floor, is entirely not recommended, since the only thing this achieves is triggering the myostatic reflex (see Introduction) and negatively affects the progress of the stretch.

The advantage of stretching the adductors with the knees flexed is that we avoid having the ischiotibial muscles intervene (as occurs in exercise 17, for example). If one wants the help of a partner, he or she may stand behind you and press with the legs, but it is more comfortable the way that is explained in the next variation.

| ...ded and the other flexed | 20.4 ... With one knee extended and the other one semi-extended |

...rting from the same position ...in the main exercise, extend ...e leg to the front and lower ...body slowly toward it. The ...erence in this variation is ...t now you are also involving ...ischiotibial muscles of the ...ended leg.

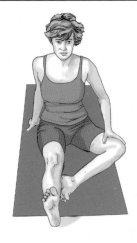

The little adage of not flexing completely the bent leg, makes us place more emphasis on the adductor minor than in the main exercise, and a little less emphasis on the rest of the adductors. However, this idea that is defended by some trainers, does not seem to be entirely well founded, given that the flexo-extension of the knee does not significantly modify the work of the major and minor adductors, which are mono-articular (they insert in the femur), and only holds up if at the same time you change the angle of the femur with respect to the knee.

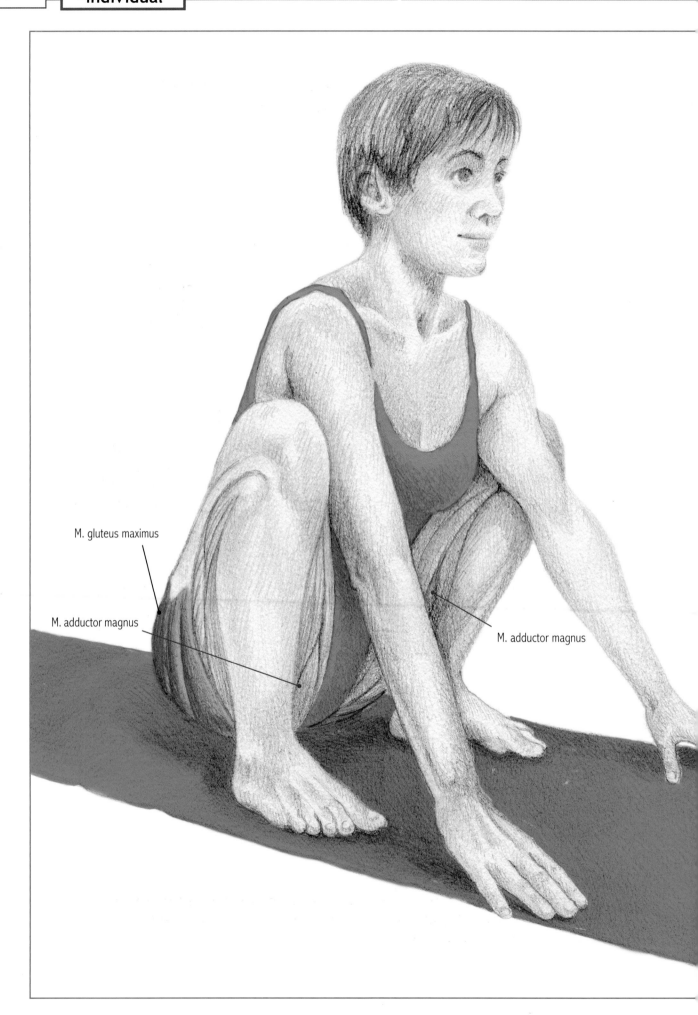

M. gluteus maximus

M. adductor magnus

M. adductor magnus